HOW TO GET PREGNANT FAST:

A complete and clinically proven guide to ovulation, conception and fertility

Dr Emma Gray

ISBN: 978-0-244-31263-3

PublishNation
www.publishnation.co.uk

Thank you Kate Davies for your thoughts on diet and supplements (http://yourfertilityjourney.com)

Important Facts to Start With

This programme is to help you to prepare both your mind and body for pregnancy and to survive the time it takes you to get to this point. The dual focus of this programme is a result of the large body of evidence that exists indicating the importance of our psychological health and balance in maintaining the optimum physical functioning of our body. It is also vital because of the intense emotional challenge of trying to conceive a baby. The pressure this put on us must be recognised and addressed if we are to hold a baby in our arms at the end of this process.

A Game of Chance [1]
The first thing to remember is that conceiving a baby is a game of chance, those that tell you that their partner only had to look at them for them to get pregnant are not more fertile than you, they have just been luckier. With the odds of conceiving in a single cycle at 20-25% for the most fertile among us (20-24 year olds), each month you roll the dice. Some of us just have to roll that dice a few more times before we hit the jackpot.

The second thing to remember is that you are more likely to get pregnant than not. Only 5% of fertile couples (i.e. those who have not been identified as infertile) will not have conceived within 2 years of trying (regardless of age). The data ends at this point so some of this group will conceive if they continue trying. This means that the longer you can stay in the game the better your chances of success.

This programme will help you to focus your energy in a helpful direction whilst you wait for your baby, it will give you control over the elements of this process that are within your control and help you to accept those that are not. And maybe, most importantly, it will give you the psychological knowledge and tools to stay in the game as long as you need to, to have your baby.

The 12 Month Pregnancy [2]

Experts say that women who are planning a pregnancy should begin preparing for it at least three months prior to actively trying to conceive. This is because it takes 3 months for immature eggs (oocytes) and sperm cells to mature, meaning the quality of the egg and sperm that develops into a baby will be dictated by your lifestyle at least 4 months before you receive a positive pregnancy test. This coupled with the fact that the greatest risk to the etus for congenital anomalies and birth defects happens between the first two to eight weeks of pregnancy has led many experts to think of pregnancy as a 12 rather than 9 month process.

This programme will help you to prepare your body and that of your partner so that the building blocks for your baby (the eggs and sperm) are of the best quality. This will not only maximise your chances of conceiving and carrying a healthy baby to term but it will also maximise your future child's physical and psychological health.

Overview

This programme covers all aspects of improving your fertility in its consideration of both the physical and emotional factors fundamental to the process of conception and a health pregnancy. It is the result of years of work with couples to overcome their fertility challenges and a thorough and comprehensive summary of the latest evidence based practice and techniques in the field of fertility. Within the two divisions of physical and emotional there are 8 sections:

1. Diet
This section includes a complete list of what foods to eat to boost fertility and why. Also, information on how to increase the nutritional profile of your food and maximise your body's ability to absorb the vitamins and minerals that will improve egg and sperm quality, support uterine health and the bodies potential to carry a healthy baby to term. It covers what foods to avoid, the importance of hydration, how to detox and how to fit all of these recommendations into your daily routine.

2. Supplements
This section includes information on to identify your individual vitamin and mineral deficiencies, a complete and comprehensive list of the supplements proven to boost fertility and specific advice for people over 35 years, those with PCOS and those with a short luteal phase.

3. Maximising Your Chances of Conception
This section includes information on how to pinpoint ovulation, scientific data on which days during your cycle to have sex to maximise your chances of conception and reduce the risk of an early miscarriage (with specific advice if you are over 35 years), medical advice regarding sexual positions and post sex routines, safeguarding sperm and improving cervical mucus. It also offers recommendations on fertility monitors.

4. Lifestyle

This section looks at the importance of a work-life balance on fertility and how to achieve this. It also considers the impact of weight, exercise, smoking and sleep on fertility and discusses the optimum parameters for each of these.

5. Alternative Approaches

This section gives an overview of Chinese Medicine (including acupuncture and Chinese herbal medicine) and how fertility problems are tackled by eastern medicine along with the scientific data that supports it. It also looks at Yoga, Fertility Massage, Reflexology, Castor Oil Therapy, Lunaception (to naturally regulate your cycle) and includes links to instructional videos to help you practice techniques at home.

6. Emotional Wellbeing

This section looks at the emotional challenges that fertility problems entail and offers practical ways of tempering and tolerating these to ensure that you can pursue your goal of having a baby without being overwhelmed by them. This section draws on a number of psychological approaches including Cognitive Behavioural Therapy (CBT) which is currently the most effective treatment for a wide range of emotional problems and challenges.

7. Miscarriage

This section looks at looks at how miscarriage is often a part of the journey to having a baby. It provides important information about prevalence, causes and ways of coping with the loss of a baby.

8. Conceiving Over 35

This section looks at the reality of trying to conceive over 35 and highlights the inaccuracies in a lot of the information that is available on this topic.

One more thing before we start.......

It can be incredibly reassuring when you are trying to conceive to know that you are doing everything you can. However, it is important that your life is not put on hold during the process as this will cause stress, resentment and frustration. These emotions will negatively impact not just on your fertility and your ability to stay in the game as long as you need to, but on other aspects of your life, ones which have the potential to bring you comfort, satisfaction and happiness. So, use this programme to tailor your own individual approach to improving your fertility, one that suits your personality and outlook but most importantly one that is sustainable. A good rule of thumb is the 80/20 rule; follow your fertility programme 80% of the time and give you self a break from it the rest of the time. This is not meant to encourage a 'bingeing' approach to those things that you are cutting out but to encourage some flexibility and self-kindness when you are faced with special occasions or just when you fancy a little treat.

Section 1: Diet

Studies have shown that a balanced healthy diet is crucial for our fertility, the better the quality of the environment the egg follicle grows in, the better the quality of the egg. This also applies to the environment that the sperm cells are developing in. In a recent survey conducted by Foresight UK[1] looking at 1,578 couples who completed their preconception programme (involving changes to diet, lifestyle and supplements), 89.8% of couples conceived and the miscarriage rate was under 3% (the national average is 25%). Most of the couples were over 33, many over 40 and some were even over 50.

So, the first step in preparing the body for a healthy pregnancy is to ensure that what you put into your body is as toxin-free and unprocessed as possible. In this section we will look in detail at how to optimise your body for pregnancy through your diet.

The 12 month pregnancy
As discussed in the introduction it is important to think of your pregnancy as a 12-month process so ideally you should make changes to your diet at least 3 months before you and your partner begin actively trying to conceive.

1. Detox

Every day we absorb heavy metals such as mercury, lead and aluminium which effect hormones and our reproductive systems. Contamination of lead and mercury in particular can cause deformities of the uterus and the fetus[2]. So it is worth considering removing these toxic substances from the body before you start the process of trying to conceive. Zeolite is a natural mineral that has been proven to remove toxins, metals and free radicals from the body. It comes in a number of different forms but the one most easily absorbed by the body is Activate Liquid Zeolite :
(http://www.liquidzeolitecompany.com/)

To support the use of Zeolite, take it alongside a diet of organic fruits and vegetables and exclude junk food so as to cleanse the body.

2. General Tips:

Try and eat foods as close to their natural state as possible.

Acidic foods can unbalance the pH level in your reproductive system which will create an inhospitable environment for sperm. So, eat plenty of non-citrus fruits, vegetables, sprouts, cereals, grasses and herbs to ensure your system stays in balance. Also, avoid alcohol and caffeine, and eat meat and dairy sparingly.

Cruciferous Vegetables like cabbage, cauliflower, broccoli, and brussels sprouts all contain the compound Di-indolylmethane (DIM), which is known to increase the metabolism of estradiol (a form of oestrogen) in the body.

Organic foods are frequently recommended by fertility experts as it is believed that they have a higher nutritional content and a lower exposure to pesticides. Recent research at Newcastle University[3] supports this to some extent but most nutritional experts stress that it is what you eat that is important, not whether it's organic or conventional. It's whether you eat fruit and vegetable at all that is going to make the biggest difference to your health and fertility.

3. Things to Include

Superfoods
For convenience and sustainability, it is worth considering preparing a smoothie each day, including in it as many superfoods as possible for both you and your partner to drink. To prevent nutrient loss eat the foods listed raw and keep your smoothie as coarse as possible, don't over blend.

Tip: If your diet has previously been high in refined carbohydrates and sugar, artificial trans fats and processed food it will take your palate a little while to adjust to a more natural, unprocessed diet. In the meantime, if your smoothie tastes a little 'sprouty' add an extra banana to temper the flavour.

Almonds contain vitamin E, which is an antioxidant that helps to protect the DNA in both sperm and eggs. Plus it's thought to increase sperm production. Almonds have been a symbol of fertility throughout the ages.

Avocados contain monounsaturated fats thought to lower inflammation in the body and therefore improve female fertility. A study measuring the diets of women undergoing IVF[4] showed that those on a diet high on the fats found in avocados were 3.4 times more likely to get pregnant.

Asparagus is filled with folic acid which has been found to reduce the risk of ovulation issues. Research studies[5] conducted on animals have demonstrated positive effects on the genitals and mammary glands of the female subjects who consumed adequate amounts of asparagus.

Bananas are packed with vitamin B6, which regulates hormones and is needed for good egg and sperm development.

Blueberries and raspberries are packed with antioxidants which help prevent damage and aging to your body's cells, including the cells in your reproductive system and egg cells. So, a diet that's rich in berries may help keep your eggs healthy and increase their shelf life.

Brussel Sprouts and Carrots contain folic acid which is great for improving fertility, they are also filled with vitamins and nutrients that help women absorb balanced levels of oestrogen and help the body get rid of excess hormones.

Cinnamon may help jump-start irregular menstrual cycles in women affected by PCOS according to preliminary research from the United States[6]. The study found that women with polycystic ovarian syndrome who took daily cinnamon supplements experienced nearly twice the menstrual cycles over a six-month period as women with the syndrome given an inactive placebo. Additionally, two of the women in the treated group reported spontaneous pregnancies during the trial.

Citrus fruits are packed with Vitamin C which improves sperm quality and stops them clumping together.

Maca has been scientifically researched [7] for the use of increasing fertility since 1961 and has been shown to contain a specific compound called glucosinolates which support hormonal balance in both men and women. It is available in powder, capsules or tincture and the powder has a malty flavour so goes well in a smoothie. Maca is particularly recommended for those with PCOS.

Pumpkin seeds are packed with zinc, the most important mineral for male and female fertility.

Tomatoes are full of a lycopene [8], a nutrient which has been found to boost sperm count by up to 70 percent.

Walnuts [9] contain potassium, phosphorus, calcium, magnesium, iron, sodium, zinc, copper, selenium, and manganese. As well as vitamins A, B1, B2, B6, B12, folate, Vitamin E and omega 3. Research has found that walnuts can significantly improve sperm vitality, motility, morphology and cause a decrease in sex chromosome disomy and sperm missing a sex chromosome.

Proteins
Protein is the building block for cellular growth and we need it to build and repair body tissues, create new cells and produce hormones. A lack of protein is considered one of the major dietary factors contributing to infertility.

According to a recent study [10] you should aim for 25 to 35 % protein intake and consume less than 40% carbohydrates per day. A free nutrition app, MyFitnessPal (www.myfitnesspal.com) will calculate the balance of nutrition in your diet and conveniently display this calculation using a pie chart so you can monitor your daily intake of fat, protein and carbs and make any necessary adjustments.

Eggs provide the perfect balance of fats and high-quality protein. They're packed with vitamin D and B6 which help boost the production of progesterone, a hormone necessary for pregnancy. They are also rich in Choline which is thought to prevent birth defects. You can eat eggs every day and an easy way to do this is by adding a raw egg to your superfoods smoothie.

Plant proteins include quinoa, beans, lentils of all types and chickpeas. There is evidence [11b] that a diet rich in plant-based sources of protein can greatly reduce the risk of ovulatory infertility. Some experts recommend they make up 50% of your plate. A word of caution here regarding soya protein as it can unbalance estrogen levels [11a].

Nuts and Seeds are a good source of healthy fat and also provide selenium and vitamin E, both of which are great for increased sperm quality and motility. Brazil nuts are an especially good source of selenium, one nut provides your daily recommended requirement. Chia seeds are considered to be the highest plant-based source of omegas, protein and fibre.

Lean protein such as lean turkey, chicken, and beef are full of iron and studies [12] show that there is a link between iron and fertility. Women who have enough iron have a higher fertility rate than women who are deficient in the nutrient. The recommended intake when trying to conceive is one serving a day. However, avoid high-fat varieties and more than three daily servings since research shows that too much protein (even lean protein) can decrease fertility.

Zinc has an important role in male fertility due to its involvement in the production of testosterone and sperm. Meat, although high in zinc, has been linked to reduced sperm quality [13] if eaten often, another reason to opt for plant-based proteins.

Liver is exponentially higher in fat soluble vitamins (A, D, E, K) and B vitamins (especially vitamin B12) as well as important minerals and fats when compared to muscle meat and produce. You can buy liver supplements if you don't like the idea of eating liver in its natural state.

Fatty fish (e.g. salmon, sardines, and herring) [14, 15] and the omega-3 fatty acids found in them are thought to regulate reproductive hormones and increase blood flow to reproductive organs. They will also keep your partner's cholesterol levels low allowing his sperm to mature properly. You can get omega-3 fatty acids from other foods such as flaxseed, walnuts, pumpkin seeds, and enriched eggs.

Carbohydrates [16a,b,c]
Carbohydrates are macronutrients in foods that provide energy to your body and include sugars, starches and fibre. However, the type of carbohydrate you eat will impact on your health and therefore your ability to conceive.

Refined Carbohydrates are processed grain that have been stripped of all their goodness (e.g. bran, germ and nutrients including 50 percent of the B vitamins, 90 percent of vitamin E and almost all of the fibre content) to increase their shelf life and make them easier to chew and digest. When eaten, refined carbohydrates are quickly broken down into simple sugars and absorbed into the blood stream causing risky spikes in insulin levels which can disrupt reproductive hormones and interfere with the menstrual cycle. For women with PCOS refined carbohydrates can lead to insulin resistance which in turns results in hormone imbalance.

Examples of refined carbohydrates:
- anything that comes in a box, bag or packet; crisps, biscuits etc.
- anything made with white flour: bread, pasta, cakes
- white rice
- sugary drinks

Unrefined Carbohydrates are a nutrient-dense food that contains high concentrations of vitamins, minerals, antioxidants and fibre. They take longer to digest and don't cause spikes in insulin levels. They also contain folic acid which increases fertility and decreases the incidence of neural-tube defects in a fetus which can occur early in pregnancy. It is also thought that unrefined carbs may promote regular ovulation.

Examples of unrefined carbohydrates:
- whole wheat or multigrain bread
- brown rice
- bran cereal
- oatmeal

Fats

Fat is vital to healthy fertility. We need a certain amount of saturated fats to produce cholesterol. Cholesterol is needed for the formation of healthy cell membranes and is a precursor to all steroid hormones (progesterone, oestrogen, FSH, etc.). We cannot have proper hormonal balance without adequate amounts of saturated fats. We cannot conceive a child or have a healthy pregnancy without proper hormonal balance.

Body fat and consumption of good fats is essential for the body to manufacture hormones and maintain hormonal balance. One study [17] showed that underweight women were 72% more likely to miscarry. On the flip side, women who are overweight may have problems conceiving due to oestrogen dominance, which may cause menstrual cycle irregularities, anovulation and inadequate building of the lining of the uterus [18].

Coconut oil is a saturate fat but it is naturally pure, healthy and is stable at high temperatures (i.e. it does not oxidise and thus expose the body to oxidative stress). Coconut oil has been shown to support adequate fat stores and help women lose weight by supporting a healthy metabolism, while balancing hormones. Whether you are at a healthy weight, low body weight or overweight, coconut oil has been shown to support a healthy metabolism by nourishing the thyroid gland [19, 20]. Metabolism and hormonal balance go hand-in-hand and coconut oil can help to support both.

Dairy

There is some debate here. Western doctors have traditionally recommended only low-fat dairy products which have beneficial protein and calcium, in order to keep weight down and insulin levels in check. Recently however many sensational headlines about eating full-fat ice cream to trigger ovulation have confused things [21].

Chinese medicine experts [22] recommend that women limit dairy intake or cut it out altogether as most dairy products contain high levels of hormones (injected into cows to produce more milk), pesticides (used in animal feed) and antibiotics which can disrupt hormones and unbalance fertility. Our digestive system is not designed to process dairy (we are the only species that drink the milk of other species) and as a result many of us have an undiagnosed dairy intolerance. Intestinal disturbance and allergies interrupt proper endocrine function and cause a thickening of cervical mucus, resulting in decreased sperm transportation, fertilization, and embryo implantation.

An approach to dairy which takes into account all of the above is as follows:

- Have a maximum of 2 servings of organic dairy each day
- If you have 2 servings per day make one serving full-fat, one low fat.
- If you only have one serving of dairy per day make it full-fat and organic
- If you go for the ice cream you may have a maximum of 1 serving of full-fat ice cream per week
- Avoid all butter! It is not a good source of fat. It can wreak havoc on your fertility by clogging up your arteries and decreasing your circulation.

Remember serving sizes are very small: 1 serving is the equivalent of 8 ounces of milk or yogurt or 1 to 1.5 ounces of cheese (1.5 oz of cheese is the size of 3 stacked dice)

Good alternatives to dairy products include milk made from seeds or nuts, such as sesame seeds, almonds, pumpkin seeds, etc. (excluding cashews and peanuts). You can also find calcium in leafy greens, canned salmon with bones, tofu, almonds, and fortified juices. Aim for about 1,000 mg of calcium daily. Soy products can also serve as an alternative but should be consumed sparingly because excessive consumption has been linked to thyroid problems [23].

If you are over 40: Studies from the US show that women who ate skimmed milk products including low-fat cheeses and yoghurts went on to delay the onset of menopause by over three-and-a-half years.

Scientists believe cow's milk may contain a number of enzymes possibly formed during the process to remove the fat, which can boost the amount of the female sex hormone oestrogen in a woman's system, helping to keep her reproductive organs working for longer [24].

Other fertility foods
Garlic contains allicin which improves blood flow to the male sex organs and protects sperm from damage, as well as selenium, an antioxidant that improves sperm quality [25].

Chocolate contains amino acid that has been proven to double sperm, increase semen volume and is filled with antioxidants which defend against free radicals and toxins linked to male infertility [26a]. Research also suggests that chocolate may be particularly good for both gestational hypertension and preeclampsia [26b].

However, the type and quality of the chocolate is very important, look for 'pure' chocolate or Cacao (available as powder or nibs) as this has undergone minimal processing so has retained maximum antioxidants. Cacao also contains no caffeine (which is often added to chocolate products and should be limited when trying to conceive), instead it contains a related stimulant called theobromine which has a similar structure to caffeine but is a very different chemical with different properties, effects and origins, it also has a beneficial impact on heart muscles and blood vessels.

Bone Broth contains minerals in a form the body can absorb easily; calcium, magnesium, phosphorus, silicon, sulphur and trace minerals. It also contains the broken down material from cartilage and tendons including chondroitin sulphates and glucosamine. Bone Broth has a range of health benefits but of particular importance for fertility it heals the gut and supports digestion which is pivotal in fertility. It is also thought to fight inflammation which is the root cause of most disease including infertility [27].
(Recipe: https://tinyurl.com/y7eblxll)

Tea contains polyphenols which prevent the chromosomal problems that can keep the egg from implanting in the uterus [28]. Green tea has half the caffeine and 10 times the polyphenols of black tea.

4. Hydration

There is a link between water consumption and fertility [29,30,31]:

- Dehydration reduces the rate of blood flow which can result in a low oxygen concentration within cells. If this continues egg cells can be damaged or malformed.
- Water helps to flush out toxins from the body. If these toxins are left to hang around they can cause stress to the reproductive system making it harder to get pregnant.
- Staying hydrated improves the quality of cervical mucus. This is essential for keeping sperm cells alive for longer and assisting them in reaching the egg.
- Water helps to deliver hormones throughout the body. Dehydration can result in a hormone imbalance, which can cause infertility.

- Chronic dehydration can cause stress, which in turn can have a negative effect on fertility.
- Dehydration can lead to reduced semen production and/or a lower sperm count
- It's important to ensure that the quality of the water you drink is high. Water straight out of the tap can contain a number of things that affect your fertility: residues from cleaning products

Bottled water is not necessarily safe as chemicals can leak out of the plastic bottles and into the water during storage. Some bottled water is also just branded tap water.

To make sure that the water you drink is clean and free of impurities it is best to invest in a good quality table-top water filter. A good example is Brita 10-Cup Everyday Water Filter Pitcher as it reduces chlorine taste and odour, zinc taste, copper, mercury and cadmium.

The European Food Safety Authority Recommendations
Women: 1.6 litres of fluid or eight 200ml glasses per day
Men: 2.0 litres of fluid or ten 200ml glasses per day

Tip: It is best to drink most of your daily fluid requirement in between meals as drinking with a meal can interfere with digestion and therefore the absorption of important nutrients. Ideally mealtime fluids should be warm and limited to a teacup full.

5. Things to Avoid

Trans fats
Researchers have found that the more trans fats in a woman's diet the greater her likelihood of developing ovulatory infertility [32]. Trans fats (also called hydrogenated or partially hydrogenated oils) are found in processed and fried foods. Read nutrition labels carefully to avoid trans fats and stick to polyunsaturated fats (in fatty fish, walnuts, and sunflower seeds) and monounsaturated fats (such as olive oil).

Caffeine

Experts say that drinking more than five cups of coffee a day (about 500 milligrams of caffeine) is associated with lower fertility [33]. To avoid a negative impact on fertility do not drink more than 200-250 milligrams (1-2 cups) of caffeine per day. For more specific guidance on how much caffeine is safe see:
https://tinyurl.com/y9zctp6s

Alcohol

Women:

Studies on alcohol intake and women's fertility have produced mixed findings. Here are some of the studies:

   a. Swedish researchers have found that women who drank two alcoholic beverages a day decreased their fertility by nearly 60% [34].

   b. A Danish study showed drinking between one and five drinks a week can reduce a woman's chances of conceiving and that 10 drinks or more decreases the likelihood of conception even further [35].

   c. A 2009 study at Harvard University of couples undergoing IVF showed that women who drank more than six units per week were 18% less likely to conceive while men were 14% less likely [36].

The Department of Health advises that women trying to get pregnant should avoid alcohol altogether. If you choose to drink the recommendations are the same as for pregnant women; 1-2 units, once or twice a week and avoid getting intoxicated.

Men:

Research suggests that men who exceed three to four units a day may damage their sperm [37].

17

Xenoestrogens

Xenoestrogens are an industrially made compound that imitates oestrogen and negatively influences the reproductive system and fertility [38]. To minimise exposure:

- Avoid processed, packaged foods and eat primarily fresh whole and preferably organic foods
- Store food in glass containers, if you cover food with plastic wrap don't let it touch the food
- Never microwave or heat food in a plastic container
- Canned foods are lined with Bisphenol, so transfer to glass containers
- Drink filtered water and bottle water from glass not plastic bottles
- Use tampons/sanitary napkins that are made of organic cotton and are free of chlorine
- Use non-bleached coffee filters
- Use detergents, soaps and shampoo that are "eco-friendly"
- Avoid all conventional pesticides, lawn and garden chemicals
- Use protective clothing when using glues, solvents and cleaning solutions
- Buy cosmetics without phthalates (also known as xenohormone)
- Avoid plug in air fresheners and diffusers

High-mercury fish

Mercury has been linked with infertility so avoid eating any high-mercury fish while trying to conceive, especially swordfish, king mackerel, tilefish, tuna steak, and shark [39].

Gluten

Data suggests that 2.6-8% of those struggling with infertility have undiagnosed celiac disease. Up to 87.5% of those with celiac disease do not have any gastrointestinal symptoms leading to a "silent" pathology that often causes decades of malaise before diagnosis. Sticking to dietary recommendations results in decreased secondary amenorrhea, delays in period onset, early menopause, and miscarriage according to a study that analysed the health of Celiac patients who adhered to a gluten free diet and those that didn't. According to data that suggests a 2.25 fold increased risk of miscarriage, intrauterine growth restriction, low birth weight, and preterm birth, this dietary change may also protect the pregnancy once it does occur [40,41,42].

6. Fermented Foods [43,44,45]

Fermentation is the process of exposing food to bacteria and yeasts, with a "starter culture" or naturally via contact with the air, to alter its properties. Historically it was to enhance taste and texture and to extend life span, but the probiotics in fermented foods also do a number of things that enhance health, including:

- Making vitamins and minerals easier to absorb, thus increasing the nutritional profile of foods
- Creating vitamins and antioxidants
- Killing off bad bacteria and yeast
- Aiding the physical and chemical digestion of food
- Making the immune system more effective and efficient

Digestive health (or 'gut flora') is the foundation of healthy fertility and is important for healing existing fertility problems. Low gut flora gives rise to inflammatory disease, a common element in endometriosis, PCOS, uterine fibroids, adenomyosis, dysmenorrhea (painful menstruation), Hashimoto's thyroiditis and autoimmune related infertility issues. Inadequate levels of gut flora also give rise to yeast infections.

Fermented foods are easy to make and some ideas are outlined below. However, you can also buy them from health food shops and some supermarkets, here are some things to consider if you plan to do this:

- Fermented foods are full of live organisms that must be kept cool to survive so only buy fermented items in the refrigerated section of the shop.
- Fermented foods will have the phrase "fermented" printed somewhere on the label.
- Be sure the label *does not* say "pasteurized", the pasteurization process wipes out the cultures you need to help fortify your gut.
- Pickled foods are not fermented.
- Look for fermented foods that are made from the best raw materials possible e.g. organic, non-GM or locally farmed produce.

Easy to Make Fermented Foods:

Sauerkraut: fermented cabbage.
Recipe:
https://tinyurl.com/yarjuw63

Kombucha tea: fermented sweet tea
Recipe:
https://tinyurl.com/3a9op8

Kefir: Similar to yoghurt this is a fizzy, tangy milk product.
Recipe:
https://tinyurl.com/2kegh9

Section 2: Supplements

It is best to get vitamins and minerals from food as it contains thousands of phytochemicals and fibre that works together to promote good health, a process that cannot be duplicated with a pill. However, even the best diet in the world may not contain all the nutrients you need to maximise your chances of conceiving and there is now a substantial body of evidence supporting the use of nutritional supplements in re-balancing hormones, eliminating nutritional deficiencies and improving sperm production and mobility.

Although supplements can support fertility they can unbalance things, so before taking large doses of vitamins try to enhance your fertility through your diet for 6 months first and only take them after other fertility tests (semen analysis, HSG to test for open tubes) come back normal.

It is important not to self-prescribe supplements (particularly if fertility tests are abnormal) but if you don't have access to a practitioner who can individually tailor a supplementation programme for you a good way of identifying vitamin and mineral deficiencies is through hair analysis. Foresight is a company that have been testing hair to restore natural fertility for over 30 years: https://tinyurl.com/yacfn87k

Once you are pregnant stop all supplements apart from a specially formulated prenatal supplement e.g Vital Essence, which offer a different formulation for the 3 different trimesters: https://tinyurl.com/y9gpoe25

Supplements to consider (doses are daily):
Note: Supplement appear in A to Z order not in order of importance

Aspirin (75-80mgs)

A daily low dose of aspirin (formerly called baby aspirin) is thought to help to increase the flow of blood to the ovaries, the uterus, improve the quality of the egg and make the uterine lining healthier, thereby helping with implantation (all of which are sometimes a problem for women over 35).

In a randomized, double-blind placebo-controlled study, 149 patients went through IVF cycles, with the only difference being the use of one low dose aspirin a day in one group and placebo in the other. Patients in the aspirin group did much better than those on the placebo. Statistically, they had more eggs, higher oestrogen levels, more uterine and ovarian blood flow, and almost double the implantation and pregnancy rates of the placebo group [1]. Some studies also suggest that for women who have miscarried frequently with no known cause, treatment with low dose aspirin can improve the chance of successful pregnancy [2].

Doctors will usually tell you to stop taking the baby aspirin after the first trimester as it can interfere with the baby's blood flow.

B-complex [3],

This family of vitamins that are necessary to produce the genetic materials DNA and RNA, not only of the egg but also the sperm and so are thought to be essential during the pre-conception period. Research has shown that giving B6 to women who have trouble conceiving increases fertility and vitamin B12 has been found to improve low sperm counts, although further human studies are necessary to determine definite benefits [4].

Beta-Carotene

Beta-carotene is a powerful antioxidant which helps to protect egg and sperm DNA from damage by harmful free radicals [5,6].

Vitamin C: 750mgs [3]

According to a study published in Fertility and Sterility [7] a moderate amount of supplemental vitamin C improves hormone levels and increases fertility. 150 women with luteal phase defect were enrolled in the study and the participants were given 750mg of vitamin C per day or no treatment at all. The group receiving vitamin C had an increase in progesterone levels, while the women receiving no treatment had no change in progesterone. In addition, the pregnancy rate was significantly higher in the vitamin C group; 25% within six months, while only 11% of the untreated women became pregnant in the same time period.

Vitamin C also enhances sperm quality, it is thought, by protecting the sperm's DNA. It also appears to keep the sperm from clumping together, making them more motile [8].

Colostrum
Colostrum is effective in supporting the immune system and has been found to be very effective for autoimmune disorders typical among women with infertility issues [9a].

Vitamin D
Research here is sparse but recent research has identified that many women suffering from infertility are also deficient in vitamin D [9b]. So particularly in countries with a less sunny climate (e.g. UK) it may be worth supplementing with this vitamin.

DHA (Docosahexaenoic acid)[3]
It is thought by some experts that DHA will become as important as Folic Acid for preconception and pregnancy. DHA is an omega-3 fatty acid and is beneficial for neurological health, the central nervous system and optical development of a fetus. While it's not always included in prenatal supplements, it is highly recommended that both pregnant and breastfeeding women take a DHA supplement. DHA can be found in appropriate quantities in fermented cod liver oil (see below).

Vitamin E [3,10,11]
Vitamin E is another powerful antioxidant and has been shown to increase fertility in both men and women. An increase from 19 to 29% in fertilisation rates has been found when this vitamin was taken by men undergoing IVF treatment with their partners.

Folic Acid: 400mgs *[3,12]*

It is now known that folic acid can prevent spina bifida in your baby so it is essential that you get plenty both before and during pregnancy. Together with vitamin B12, folic acid also works to ensure that your baby's genetic codes are intact.

Folic acid may however not be the best option for those with MTHFR mutations in these cases. For more information: https://tinyurl.com/yal3s6ut

L-Arginine: 300mgs *[13]*

L-arginine is thought to improve the reproductive health of both men and women because:

- It increases blood circulation to the uterus, ovaries and genitals which will improve egg production, improve the chances of conception and create a better environment for implantation.
- It increases nitric oxide levels which research has found supports healthy inflammation levels that may help to prevent uterine fertility issues such as fibroids, endometriosis and PCOS.
- It supports normal sperm production; research has found that taking an l-arginine supplement daily can increase sperm production in men and may also improve the motility of sperm, thus increasing the chance of conception in couples suffering from low sperm motility. Where IVF is used, l-arginine can be used to improve the quality of sperm, increasing the chance of achieving a fertilized egg.
- It improves the production of cervical mucous by increasing blood flow to the reproductive organs.
- It supports a healthy libido by increasing blood flow to the genitals in both men and women. In men, increased blood flow to the penis can result in more frequent and sustained erections. L-arginine is often suggested for men suffering from erectile dysfunction. In women, increased blood flow

to the genitals can lead to increased sexual arousal and orgasm.

Note: People who have herpes attacks (either cold sores or genital herpes) should not supplement with L-arginine because it stimulates the virus.

L-Carnitine: *100mgs [14,15]*
This amino acid is essential for normal functioning of sperm cells. According to research it appears that the higher the levels of L-Carnitine in the sperm cells, the better the sperm count and motility.

Omega Fatty Acids [16,17,18]
These essential fats are crucial for healthy hormone functioning and control inflammation which may interfere with getting and staying pregnant. In addition, semen is rich in prostaglandins (inadequate levels result in poor sperm quality, motility and count) which are produced from these fats. Research has shown that men and women with higher levels of blood omega-3 fatty acids have increased fertility rates compared to people with lower levels of blood omega-3 fatty acids. It is important that the supplement that you take has a high DHA:EPA ratio. A good example is Fermented Cod Liver Oil (a natural source of Omega 3,6,7, & 9 and vitamins A & D) which unlike most fish oil supplements has not been heat treated (which destroys naturally occurring vitamin A and D content and denatures the delicate omega-3 fatty acids) making the nutrient content and delicate fatty acids much more bio-available to our bodies.

PABA - 300 to 400 mg
PABA is the short name of Para-aminobenzoic acid and is classified as a vitamin like substance. It is commonly known as an antioxidant and a micronutrient. PABA can be naturally found in a variety of food; from spinach and mushrooms to brewer's yeast and wheat germ. Although it is not a true vitamin, it is often referred to be as vitamin Bx. When PABA is consumed it helps stimulate the pituitary gland which proves to be a useful element for women who have trouble in conceiving. It also has a positive impact on the formation of red blood cells which stimulates the production of folic acid in the

intestines. A clinical trial in 1942 reported that after supplementing with PABA over several months 12 out of 16 infertile women became pregnant [19].

Selenium: 100mgs [3]
Selenium helps to protect your body from free radicals and therefore can prevent chromosome breakage, a cause of birth defects and miscarriages. Selenium is also essential to maximise sperm formation. Selenium levels have been found to be lower in men with low sperm counts [20a].

However, some experts advise caution when using Selenium as it may strip the sperm of its oxidation (which is necessary for healthy sperm production). Instead they suggest supplementing with Condensyl [20b,c].

Zinc: 30mgs [21,22]
Zinc is an essential component of genetic material and the most widely studied fertility nutrient for both men and women. Zinc is necessary for your body to efficiently use the reproductive hormones, oestrogen and progesterone. A zinc deficiency can cause chromosome changes in either you or your partner, leading to reduced fertility and an increased risk of miscarriage.

Zinc is also needed to make the outer layer and tail of the sperm and is therefore, essential for the health of your partner's sperm. Several studies have also shown that reducing zinc in a man's diet will also reduce his sperm count.

For Women Over 35

CoQ-10: 600 milligrams per day [23,24,25]
Ovulation involves a long process of cell development and Co-enzyme Q10 is essential in cell development, as we get older our bodies produce less CoQ-10. Current advice is extrapolated from animal studies but experts suggest that taking up to 600 milligrams a day of Co-enzyme Q10 may help to improve egg quality in older women and improve fertilization. This is a relatively inexpensive

supplement and there is no risk attached to taking it as CoQ-10 occurs naturally in the body.

Studies have also found that Co-enzyme Q10 may also improve male infertility. A July 2009 study in *The Journal of Urology* looked at 212 infertile men who took 300 mg of the supplement for 30 weeks, and found that it improved both sperm density and motility.

DHEA (micronized): 3 x 75mgs per day [26]
DHEA is a naturally occurring hormone that the female body converts into androgens, mainly testosterone. Even though androgens are male hormones they're present in both sexes and are essential in the female body for the production and development of healthy eggs. The Centre for Human Reproduction (CHR) (New York) has conducted a number of studies looking at the impact of this supplement and have concluded the following:

1. DHEA supplementation improves IVF pregnancy rates and shortens time to pregnancy.
2. DHEA increases the chance of spontaneous pregnancies.
3. DHEA supplementation improves the quality and quantity of eggs and embryos.
4. DHEA reduces chromosomal abnormalities in embryos, resulting in a lower risk of miscarriages.
5. DHEA also improves cumulative pregnancy rates in patients undergoing fertility treatment.

DHEA is used to treat women with diminished ovarian reserve (DOR), which occurs either as a consequence of premature ovarian aging (POA) or female aging. If you fall into one of these groups and are interested in taking DHEA you can read more by following the link:
https://tinyurl.com/y7ohvmxq

Note: DHEA should only be taken in consultation with a medical practitioner who can monitor dosage levels.

Note: DHEA must be in a micronized form so that the body can absorb it.

Note: Women with PCOS have elevated levels of androgens and so should not take DHEA as it will acerbate two side effects of PCOS; acne and unwanted hair growth.

Melatonin: 3mgs [27]
Melatonin is best known for its ability to treat insomnia and jet-lag. It is a potent antioxidant and seems to protect the cell's sensitive genetic material (DNA) from being damaged. Melatonin, a natural hormone that the body produces, may be helpful in women with poor quality eggs. Experts speculate that it works by protecting the egg against oxidative damage. Moreover, low melatonin levels seem to impair sperm motility in men. Melatonin can be taken as a supplement or found in the following foods: pineapples, bananas, oranges, tomatoes, sweetcorn, and sour cherry juice.

For PCOS

Black Cohosh: 120 milligrams per day for first 10 day of cycle
Black Cohosh has been able to reduce the high levels of inflammatory chemicals found in those with PCOS. A recent study comparing Black Cohosh with Clomid, found that Black Cohosh resulted in significant improvements in key gonadotropin markers such as LH and LH/FSH ratios and resulted in better progesterone levels than Clomid, indicating stronger, healthier ovulation and greater chances of implantation. Although it did not reach clinical significance, the pregnancy rate was also higher in the patients who received Black Cohosh, when compared to those who received Clomid [28].

Agnus Castus (Vitex/Chastetree berry) [29]
Agnus Castus is a fertility-promoting herb with a long, safe history of human use. High quality studies are limited but preliminary findings suggest that it may help stimulate and stabilize the reproductive hormones involved in ovulation, cycle balance, and menstrual regularity.

Inositol [30]
Inositol is a vitamin-like substance that is found in many plants and animals but can also be made in a laboratory. It is thought to balance chemicals in the body to help with PCOS.

Clinical research has shown the following effects of inositol supplementation:

1. Restoration of spontaneous ovarian activity and consequently fertility in most patients with PCOS.

2. Improvement in ovarian stimulation protocols and pregnancy outcomes in infertile women with poor oocyte quality.

3. Increases in peak progesterone.

N-Acetyl Cysteine (NAC) [31]
N-Acetyl Cysteine (NAC) maintains the proper functioning of the lungs and supports the immune system and liver function. NAC is also a powerful antioxidant. It acts as a mucolytic and increases the levels of glutathione in the body. It can also be useful for insulin resistance and improving fertility. A recent study showed that NAC dramatically reduced testosterone and homocysteine levels in 6 lean and 31 obese women with PCOS.

Cinnulin PF [32]
Cinnulin PF is an aqueous cinnamon extract with a high concentration of active Type-A Polymers that have been shown to support healthy blood sugar metabolism, cholesterol management, and weight management, as well as having potent antioxidant properties. Recent studies showed that consumption of cinnamon reduced insulin resistance in 15 PCOS women and women with infertility issues.

For Short Luteal Phase
The normal range for a luteal phase is between 10-16 days i.e. anything within this is sufficient to support a pregnancy.

Vitamin B6 [33,34]: 50mg per day
Vitamin B6 has been widely studied and shown to be effective at correcting a luteal phase defect. Vitamin B6 can be found in foods such as: tuna fish, liver, bananas, salmon and many green vegetables.

There are a number of multivitamins and supplements that have been formulated to include many of the above so it may be helpful to check the ingredients against this list when making your choice. Good examples include:

1. Fertility Support for Women (also available for Men)
   https://tinyurl.com/y8orprpn

2. Fertility Blend (also available for Men)
   https://tinyurl.com/37648

3. Vitafem
   https://tinyurl.com/yd9dad9s

Natural Supplements
Currently no randomised controlled studies have been conducted investigating the effectiveness of these supplements but the following are often recommended by fertility experts:

Bee pollen and Royal Jelly
These are said to alleviate menstrual problems in women and increase sperm production in men.

Blue-Green Algae
Said to regulate metabolism and repair damaged tissues.

Wheatgrass
Used to nourish the blood, enhance immunity and restore hormonal balance.

Section 3: Maximising the Chances of Conception

The reality is that if you are having sex regularly (ideally 2 to 3 times per week) you are more likely than not to conceive within 2 years, regardless of age. However, there are a number of things that you can do to speed up this process, some of which have been validated by research, others of which remain unproven theories.

1. Timing Sex [1,2,3,4,5,6,7]
The table below outlines the chances of getting pregnant in relation to the number of days before ovulation that you have sex:

Days Before Ovulation	Chances of Conceiving
5	10%
4	16%
3	14%
2	27%
1	31%
Day of Ovulation	33%
Day after Ovulation	0%

However, research that looked at pregnancies that survived past 6 weeks found that a large percentage of conceptions from sex on the day of ovulation led to early miscarriages indicating that the best time to have sex is on days 1 and 2 before ovulation. This is probably due to the fact that the minute the egg is produced it begins to degrades, if sperm is waiting for it at the point of ovulation it is going to be fresher than if they meet it half way down your fallopian tubes.

If you are over 35....
A study from the 1990s found that sex two days before ovulation led to pregnancy among 25% of 35-39 year olds after just one cycle, the

same percentage of women aged 19-26 who got pregnant when they had sex three days before ovulation. So timing sex just one day better eliminated the age difference in fertility.

Finally, researchers at Indiana University found that having sex outside of the fertile window also increases the possibility of pregnancy. Immune changes were found in sexually active women that increased their fertility as if the body was preparing in advance for the mere possibility of pregnancy.

2. Positions [8]
Unless your cervix is in an unusual position there is no scientific evidence to support the idea that sexual position will maximise chances of conception. However, some experts do still recommend rear entry ('doggy style'), missionary and side by side as optimal positions to allow for the deepest penetration and contact with the cervix, while minimizing the chance of leakage. Other experts also suggest having your partner keep his penis inside you for as long as possible after his orgasm as this is thought to create a good barrier and keep the semen concentrated close to the cervix.

It is also thought that if a female has an orgasm after her partner, the sperm gets "sucked up" into the cervix which helps to get them where they are needed faster. However again, this is a theory that has yet to be proven.

3. After Sex
It is often suggested that after sex you should elevate your hips to assist the sperm in their journey into the cervix. However, your pelvis does not move when you do this so it is sufficient to just lie down for 10-15 minutes and allow gravity to get the sperm going in the right direction. The sperm that is going to reach the cervix will have done so in this time.

Supporting this is a study of 391 women published in the British Medical Journal in which Dutch researchers found that the pregnancy rate among women who laid down after insemination was

27%, compared to 18% for those who got straight up and moved around [9].

4. Safeguarding Sperm [10,11]
Sperm are produced every day, but they mature after 70 days. What this means is that if there is any damage to the sperm it takes more than two months for new sperm to mature and be ready to fertilize an egg. So changes to your partner's diet and lifestyle will take time at least this amount of time to have an effect.

Try to have sex at least every five days during the time you are not trying to conceive in an effort to flush out the sperm. This will ensure that you have healthy sperm when you need them. Then approximately 5 days before you will ovulate, have sex either every day or every other day up until and including the day of ovulation.

Finally, most lubricants and saliva can damage sperm so during your fertile window abstain from oral sex and if you use a lubricant use one that is sperm-friendly (e.g. Preseed: http://www.preseed.co.uk/).

5. Cervical Mucus [12,13,14]
Cervical mucus provides the environment for the sperm to travel through your vagina, your uterus, and up to the fallopian tubes where they can fertilize the egg. If your cervical mucus is too thick or acidic it can be hostile to the sperm. To maximise its quality, quantity and consistency:

- Stay hydrated
  Cervical mucus is 90% water so if you are dehydrated your cervical mucus will suffer

- Grapefruit Juice
  A glass of grapefruit juice every day during the last week before ovulation can improve the quantity and consistency of your mucus, making it thinner and easier to move through for the sperm cells. Despite being acidic, grapefruit juice has

an alkalizing effect once digested, which can help make the mucus even more sperm-friendly.

- Raw Garlic
  Some women have reported more abundant cervical mucus after eating a clove of fresh, raw garlic every day before ovulation.

- Antihistamines
  Antihistamines and decongestants will dry up your cervical mucus. If you need to use antihistamines, ask your doctor for advice on how to avoid adverse effects on your production of cervical mucus while you are trying to conceive.

- Cough syrup
  If you think your cervical mucus is too thick, expectorant cough medicine can help make it thinner. Make sure the active ingredient is *guaifenesin*, use it during the last few days before ovulation, and do not take more than the recommended daily dose indicated on the package.

- Evening Primrose Oil
  Evening Primrose Oil is a herbal supplement containing a fatty acid called GLA (Gamma Linolenic Acid). The human body converts GLA into prostaglandins, which may enhance the production of fertile cervical mucus.

- L Arginine
  L-Arginine is another supplement which may help improve cervical mucus by increasing the production of nitric oxide. Nitric oxide dilates blood vessels and helps to increase blood flow to the uterus, ovaries, and genitals.

6. Pinpointing Ovulation [15,16,17,18]
As mentioned earlier, being able to pinpoint ovulation can significantly reduce the amount of time it takes to conceive. There are 3 main strategies here:

I.   Measuring Basal Body Temperature (BBT)
Your BBT is your body's temperature at rest. When you
ovulate your body produces progesterone which creates heat
and causes a rise in your BBT. When your BBT rises by 0.2
degrees and remains high for 3 consecutive days this usually
means you have ovulated.

It is best to use a digital thermometer that reads to the tenth
place (e.g. XX.X) when measuring your BBT. You do not
need a thermometer specifically designed for the purpose but
equally do not use a traditional mercury thermometer. For an
accurate reading:

   a.   Keep your thermometer by your bed and take your
        temperature as soon as you wake and at the same
        time every morning. Eating, drinking or moving will
        all cause your temperature to rise above your BBT.

   b.   Take your temperature after at least 3 hours of
        consecutive sleep

   c.   Record your temperature on a graph

The graph below shows a typical cycle of 28 days, with the
follicular phase (i.e. prior to ovulation) beginning on day 4-5
following the completion of menses and ending at the point
of ovulation (day 15) which can be identified by the sharp
increase in BBT. The luteal phase then begins and continues
until day 28 when in the absence of fertilisation of the egg,
BBT falls and menses starts.

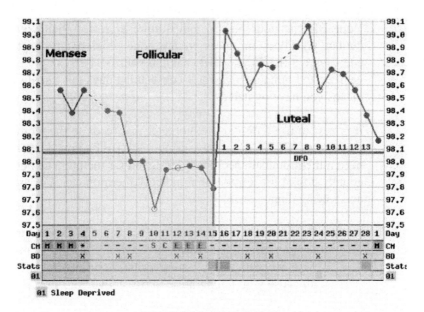

Tip 1. If you snore or sleep with your mouth open your readings will not be accurate so you will instead need to measure your core temperature (which is more accurate then BBT) using a device such as Ovusense (see below).

Tip 2. Some women experience a slight dip in their temperature prior to the rise that indicates ovulation. This usually occurs between 1-3 days before ovulation and so can be used to predict impending ovulation. Some experts however suggest that this dip is rarely seen in practice. For more information:
https://tinyurl.com/ya6p5x4d

Tip 3. Some women will notice a third rise in BBT around day 7-10 post ovulation (see graph below). This is called a triphasic shift and can indicate successful implantation of an embryo into the uterus. However, only 12% of women who are pregnant will experience a triphasic shift so don't assume you're not pregnant if you don't see it. Equally it is not a definite sign of pregnancy, progesterone levels peak at some point in the luteal phase which can results in what appears to be a triphasic shift in the absence of implantation.

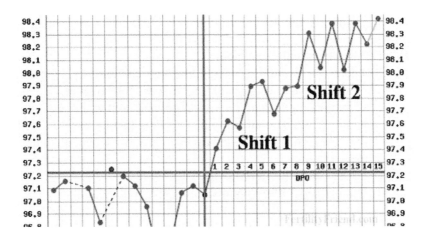

II.   Monitoring Cervical Mucus
The texture and consistency of cervical mucus changes throughout the month and can serve as a good indicator of when you will ovulate. As ovulation gets closer and your oestrogen production increases, your cervical mucus will change from a creamy texture to a clear stretchy texture (like raw egg white). Sperm can survive for several days in this fertile mucus so when you see it this is the best time to try and get pregnant. Some experts suggest that this is the most reliable indicator of impending ovulation.

Tip: When checking for cervical mucus use your fingers and not toilet paper which will absorb some of the moisture. It's also important to check the mouth of the vagina, not the walls since they are always moist.

III.   Monitoring Cervical Position
The position of your cervix can also indicate ovulation. Outside of your fertile window your cervix will feel firm, dry, easy to reach, and closed. Closer to ovulation it will become softer, wetter, open and harder to reach as it pulls further up into the uterus.

IV.   Fertility Monitors and Apps
There are a number of monitors that can assist you in pin pointing ovulation and although they cost between £300-£500 they include support packages and help you to not only predict but also confirm ovulation thus taking away a lot of the guess work and subsequent anxiety. Good examples include:
Ovusense - http://www.ovusense.com/uk/
DuoFertility - http://www.duofertility.co.uk/

Fertility Friend is a free app that allows you to record your observations of these fertility signs and compare them to your hormonal profile in order to determine your fertile window:
https://www.fertilityfriend.com/

For a useful comparison of currently available fertility apps and monitors:
https://tinyurl.com/yah63ab6

Section 4: Lifestyle

Moderation is key here, anything extreme (too much or too little) is likely to upset the natural balance of your fertility.

The Work-Life Balance
Finding a balance between the demands of work and an innate drive within all of us to achieve, whilst creating time to rest, relax and look after ourselves is an age-old challenge. Finding this balance is particularly important if you are trying to conceive because a lack of equilibrium in the way that you structure your time can lead to a whole range of problems from anxiety, depression and anger to physical health problems. All of these problems will impact not only your fertility but your capacity to manage the physical and emotional rollercoaster that trying to conceive can become.

In Psychology we talk about finding a balance between what you NEED to do and what you WANT to do. One way to evaluate this balance in your life is to use a pie chart to depict your various time commitments:

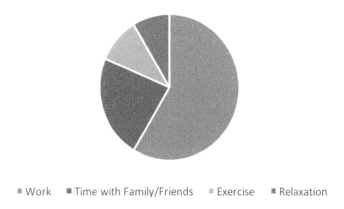

■ Work   ■ Time with Family/Friends   ■ Exercise   ■ Relaxation

Once you have done this ask yourself:

- Are you happy with what you see?

- Do you think you are achieving a healthy balance between what you NEED to do and what you WANT to do?

- Would someone else looking at this chart agree with you?

If you find an imbalance consider the short and long term consequences of not making a change by completing the table as shown below:

	Pros of Making a Change	Cons of Making a Change
Short term (days/weeks)	• A boost in mood from knowing I am making positive changes	• Time consuming • Logistical challenges • Negative reactions from others
Long term (months/years)	• Improved physical and emotional health and therefore fertility	• Need to find motivation to keep changes going

Weight

Many women in the underweight, overweight, and obese categories will not have a problem becoming pregnant. However, having a body weight outside of the normal range (Body Mass Index {BMI} = 19-25) can disrupt your hormones which in turn increases your chances of having problems with ovulation.

You can use the formula below to work out your BMI:

Weight (kgs)/Height (m2)

e.g. 58/1.6m2 = 58/2.56 = 22.6

BMI = 22.6 (normal range)

If your BMI is either less than 18 or greater than 29 you may need a combination of nutritional and psychological support to bring your weight back within the normal range. Please contact The British CBT & Counselling Service (www.thebritishcbtcounsellingservice.co.uk) for more information about how to access this support.

Exercise

Under or overweight women should seek an evaluation from a certified fitness professional to tailor a program based on their energy input and output.

Moderation again is key. Preliminary research [1] suggests that regular workouts may actually improve reproductive function: A study in *Obstetrics & Gynaecology* concluded that women who exercised for 30 minutes or more daily had a reduced risk of infertility due to ovulation disorders. On the other hand, some data [2] links too much vigorous exercise with lowered fertility. More than an hour of vigorous exercise a day can lead to a decrease in the production of the hormones that stimulate ovary function, causing ovaries to become underactive and stop producing eggs and oestrogen. In addition, over exercising causes the body to break down the proteins in muscles, producing ammonia, a pregnancy-inhibiting chemical and a shorter luteal phase has been found amongst marathon runners and professional athletes [3].

Mostly because there have been no controlled studies of exercise in women who are trying to get pregnant naturally it is recommended that women follow the Department of Health's advice regarding exercise:

1. At least 150 minutes (2 hours and 30 minutes) of moderate-intensity aerobic activity such as cycling or fast walking every week and

2. Muscle-strengthening activities on 2 or more days a week that work all major muscle groups (legs, hips, back, abdomen, chest, shoulders and arms).

Some specialists are going beyond this generic mandate and suggest if your BMI is between 20-25 (normal range) to keep workouts to an hour or less per day unless your cycle is irregular or you haven't conceived after a few months, then cut back further and don't do any exercise that raises your heart rate above 110 beats per minute [4]. Also, this is not the time to start a rigorous exercise programme if this is not what your body is used to, even if your BMI or body fat percentage stays the same the stress can have a negative effect on reproductive hormone production and fertility.

Recommendation from a Chinese Medicine Perspective [5,6,7]

- Avoid anything that puts a down-bearing pressure or strain on your uterus (e.g. weight lifting) to prevent the uterus "falling" or the lining weakening. Women with a history of miscarriage should take extra care here. Also, excessive abdominal work (like Pilates) should be minimized as this can constrict blood flow to the uterus as well as strain it.

- Avoid excessive sweating. Your fluids are crucial for the health of your fertility and even if you re-hydrate your body may become depleted of critical fluids that contribute to your fertility. Women who have light or short periods, skip periods, or have long cycles should take extra care. In this case, you're likely already fluid deficient.

- Regular exercise is great, but sometimes less is more. If your body is already exhausted and you're running on empty, excessive exercise will drain your adrenal glands. This signals to the body that it's under extreme stress. Not only will this take away from the precious energy needed to support your reproductive system, it will shut down your reproductive hormones.

Exercises in line with the above recommendations:

- Brisk walks
- Gentle to moderate stretching e.g. yoga
- Qigong and Tai Chi*
- Swimming
- Low-impact dancing
- Gentle bike rides
- Easy hikes

*This is Chinese style yoga which directs energy through the acu-channels of the body and can help to lift energy, replenish fluids and increase your qi.

Smoking and Sleeping
There are three exceptions to the moderation rule, alcohol (which is dealt with in section 1) smoking and sleeping.

1. Smoking [8,9,10]
Both active and passive smoking effects fertility. In fact passive smoking is only slightly less harmful to fertility than active smoking. Here are the key facts:

- Smokers take longer to conceive than non-smokers and are more likely to have fertility problems.

- Smoking ages your ovaries by 10 years

- Smoking is incredibly damaging to sperm

- The risk of infertility among smokers may be twice that of non-smokers.

- Women who smoke are at least 1.5 times more likely than non-smokers to take longer than a year to get pregnant. If a male partner is a heavy smoker, this will significantly contribute to delayed conception.

- Female passive smokers are more likely than women in non-smoking homes to take more than a year to get pregnant.

- Smoking women reach menopause earlier than non-smoking women.

- The more you smoke the more you risk affecting your fertility – both your ability to get pregnant and the time it takes to get pregnant.

- The good news is that most of the negative effects of smoking on fertility are reversed a year after stopping smoking.

2. Sleep *[11,12,13]*

An adequate amount of sleep is necessary to balance a number of fertility hormones including progesterone, oestrogen, luteinizing hormone (LH) and follicle-stimulating hormone (FSH). It is also crucial in the production of leptin, a hormone that affects ovulation. When leptin production is compromised, menstrual cycles are disrupted.

To protect your fertility try to get a minimum of 7 hours sleep per night. To boost your fertility aim for 8-9 hours.

Section 5: Alternative Approaches

Chinese Medicine [1,2,3,4,5]
Chinese medicine is based on observations of the human body collected over the past 2,000 years. It has always been concerned with how to slow down the ageing process and contends that the key to overall health and fertility resides with our 'Jing'.

You are born with two kinds of Jing: your pre-natal Jing (DNA), that you inherit from your parents and your post-natal Jing (energy or life-force) that you can maintain through the kind of lifestyle you choose. Chinese medicine stresses the importance of living in a way that nourishes and preserves our post-natal Jing.

Western society is plagued with all sorts of stressors (long work hours, toxins, stimulants, lack of sleep) that consume our Jing and cause us to age prematurely thereby causing our fertility to decline at an accelerated rate. In addition to making changes to your diet and lifestyle you can nourish and protect your Jing in order to slow down the ageing process and improve your fertility potential through acupuncture and herbal medicine.

Acupuncture
By placing needles at key energy meridians linked to the reproductive organs, acupuncture stimulates and restores the flow of Qi, a form of life energy that according to theories of Chinese medicine must flow through the body unhampered if illness or malfunctions such as infertility are to be avoided. A more western understanding of the process is that acupuncture increases blood supply by dilating the arteries to the ovaries so that they receive greater amounts of hormonal stimulation and to the lining of the uterus so that it is better able to absorb the nutrients and hormones necessary to help it grow strong enough to hold onto an implanted embryo. To function at peak capacity, both the ovaries and the uterus must have adequate blood supply, poor blood flow can inhibit

pregnancy. Acupuncture is currently the only proven technique able to directly increase vascular response [6].

Research has concluded that acupuncture: [7,8,9,10]

- increases production of endorphins that play a role in regulating the menstrual cycle.

- has a neuroendocrine effect, impacting a three-way axis between the two areas of the brain involved with hormone production (the hypothalamus and the pituitary glands) and the ovaries, a constellation that ultimately impacts egg production and possibly ovulation.

- substantially increased pregnancy success when added to IVF treatment protocols; 34 pregnancies, compared with 21 in the women who received IVF alone.

- stimulated egg production and was as effective as Clomid

- may directly impact the number of egg follicles available for fertilization in women undergoing IVF.

To find a qualified practitioner visit The British Acupuncture Society:
http://www.acupuncture.org.uk/

Chinese Herbs
Records indicate that Chinese herbs have been used in the treatment of infertility and miscarriage since 200 A.D. However, no one herb is considered especially useful for promoting fertility, rather, more than 150 different herbs, usually given in complex formulas comprised of 15 or more ingredients, are used in the treatment of infertility with the purpose of correcting a specific functional or organic problem believed to underlie an individual's infertility.

In modern China, herbs are used to treat infertility in both men and women and the results of large scale clinical trials are reported in Chinese medical journals [11]. Results from these studies suggest:

- 70% of all cases of infertility (male and female) treated by Chinese herbs resulted in pregnancy or restored fertility.

- Depending on the particular study and the types of infertility treated, success rates ranged from about 50% up to more than 90%

- Included in these statistics are cases of infertility involving obstruction of the fallopian tubes, amenorrhea, absent ovulation, endometriosis, uterine fibroids, low sperm count, nonliquification of semen, and other causes.

To find a practitioner in Chinese Herbal Medicine visit The Register of Chinese Herbal Medicine: http://www.rchm.co.uk/

Yoga

Women who are under constant stress produce prolactin, cortisol and other hormones, which can interfere with or even block regular ovulation. Studies show that yoga can help reduce stress and bring some calmness and balance to the mind which can affect fertility [12,13,14]. Some experts [15] also believe that specific poses can help promote conception by increasing blood flow to your pelvis, stimulating hormone-producing glands, and releasing muscle tension.

Follow this link for more information and specific yoga poses: https://tinyurl.com/y9s8rzod

(Self) Fertility Massage [16,17,18]

Fertility massage has been used for hundreds of years to support conception. Some of the benefits are thought to include:

- Increasing blood circulation
- Boosting egg health by increasing oxygenated blood flow to the ovaries which are often suffocated due to an impaired ovulation cycle wherein they suffer from a lack of nutrients and oxygenated blood
- Maintaining hormonal balance
- Removing useless tissues (especially remains from previous menstruation and pelvic injuries)
- Re-positioning a tilted uterus
- Breaking down cysts in cases of polycystic ovarian syndrome
- Breaking down pelvic adhesions and stimulating blood flow to speed up recovery of scars
- Reducing pain and cramps during menstrual cycle
- Regulating menstrual cycles
- Detoxifying and encouraging the liver to detoxify and mop out excess hormones
- Reducing clotting during menstrual cycle
- Eliminating bloating and water retention in the reproductive system area
- Relieving the uterus area of old stagnant blood and bringing in fresh blood
- Strengthening the reproductive organs
- Preparing muscles for child birthing
- Clearing the fallopian tubes for unhindered movement of egg and sperm
- Improving digestion and getting rid of discomfort in the abdominal region
- Promoting relaxation

The best time to practice (self) fertility massage is between days 6-14 of your cycle as it can help ensure a regular supply of oxygenated blood and the distribution of hormone towards the reproductive area while the egg is being developed and released. Avoid fertility massage during the time that you are menstruating as fertility massage may increase your blood flow and also during your luteal phase to ensure that you don't interfere with implantation.

Femoral Reproductive Massage
This type of massage increases the blood flow to the pelvic area providing extra nourishment to the uterus and ovaries. This video gives more specific information, a demonstration of the technique and how to do it yourself:
https://tinyurl.com/y7aomdns

Acupressure Abdominal Massage
Acupressure is an alternative therapy that is easy, effective, and can be done at home to help improve fertility. Acupressure has been applied for thousands of years to help improve hormonal balance, the menstrual cycle and aid conception. Acupressure comes from Traditional Chinese Medicine, based on the same ideas as acupuncture, but without the needles. It involves applying pressure with the fingers to specific points on the body. The stimulation of these points signal the body to increase circulation and energy to another area of the body. This video demonstrates an easy acupressure massage that can be incorporated into a self-fertility massage routine.
https://tinyurl.com/ybon55wr

Fertility Massage
The following protocol incorporates all of the above techniques:

1. Lie down with your back on a mat, bench or even a hard surface.

2. Place a towel under your head and a pillow under your lumbar region (i.e. containing the 5 vertebrae that form the curve in the back).

3. Start with the Femoral Reproductive Massage Technique.

4. Get some massage oil on your hands and warm up your fingers.

5. Press gently on your uterus and work your way up and down, from the pubic bone to the navel and back.

6. Press on the uterus and try pulling it up towards the navel. Hold the uterus in this position for a few seconds or to the count of 10. Repeat this exercise up to 15 times.

7. Perform the Acupressure Abdominal Massage.

8. Massage your whole tummy with a clockwise circular motion starting from the navel until it covers the whole stomach.

9. End the massage with another round of Femoral Reproductive Massage Technique.

Further Information
It you would like to explore this area further Hethir Rodriguez, a certified massage therapist and a master herbalist has created a natural fertility therapy to help women apply the fertility massage techniques for themselves and called it Self Fertility Massage™.

Self Fertility Massage™ comprises a wide range of massage techniques such as Chi Nei Tsang (Asian organ massage), deep tissue massage, myofascial release, acupressure, reflexology and castor oil therapy. For more information:
https://tinyurl.com/ybon55wr

Reflexology
Reflexology works to bring the body into a state of balance, encouraging the body's systems to work to their optimum level to create a healthier environment for pregnancy to occur.

A randomised controlled research trial [19] looking at the effectiveness of reflexology in ovulation induction is currently ongoing at Derriford Hospital Plymouth and the complementary medicine department at the University of Exeter and has been extended to include Exeter's Fertility Unit and University College Hospital Fertility Unit, London. The number of pregnancies to date total 30.

This video shows you the areas of the feet that are manipulated during reflexology so you can try the techniques yourself: https://www.youtube.com/watch?v=B_NJxp5Wogs

Castor oil packs [20,21]
Castor oil therapy has been used for centuries to promote healing in the body and more specifically the reproductive system. By applying a castor oil pack externally, positive benefits have been found including:

- Supporting ovarian health
- Supporting fallopian tube health
- Supporting uterine health
- Detoxifying before conception
- Supporting egg health

Castor oil packs stimulate 3 important parts of the body: lymphatic and circulatory systems and the liver. The stimulation of these body systems aids the body in healing the organs and tissues beneath where the castor oil pack is applied. Follow this link to find out how to do this at home:
https://tinyurl.com/y7y778yw

Lunaception [22,23,24]
Lunaception is the practice of balancing hormones by controlling the light in the room where we sleep. Much of our hormone production is done at night and light in the room signals their release. It is suggested that before electricity most women experienced their menstrual cycles with the phases of the moon and at more or less the same time as all other women, ovulating at the full moon and menstruating at the new moon.

Lunaception uses light to control ovulation. The recommendation is that all light be excluded from the bedroom at night, except during the three fullest days of the moon (the day of the full moon and the days preceding and following), when a small light should shine throughout the night. It is claimed that after several months, the menstrual cycle should come into balance with the light and as a result your body can obtain a greater level of reproductivity. When attempting to conceive, intercourse is recommended on those three nights when the moon is fullest because according to the theory, we should ovulate during a full moon and menstruate with a new moon.

While not scientifically proven, the theory offers an alternative for women to regulate their cycles and predict their fertility and is supported by significant anecdotal reports of success.

What you need to do:

For irregular cycles
Sleep in complete darkness starting at the new moon. This means after 15 minutes you cannot see your hand in front of your face. Using an eye mask is not sufficient as light can enter the body through other openings (e.g. ears and nostrils). If you often get up at night to use the bathroom place dim nightlights in the hallway and bathroom, do not turn on overhead lights.

The day before the full moon, allow a small amount of light into the room. Natural moon light through a window is best, otherwise try and find a very white, yet dim nightlight for your room.

Three days later go back to sleeping in complete darkness until the next full moon.

For regular or semi-regular cycle
Mark the first day of your last period as day one.

From day 14 -16 sleep with a small amount of light in the room.

Following this go back to sleeping in complete darkness.

If you have a 28-30 day cycle keep following your cycle and on days 14-16 sleep with a small amount of light in the room.

If you have a long cycle on day 30, even if your period starts, start numbering again at one and sleep in light on days 14-16 again.

Section 6: Emotional Wellbeing

The emotional challenge of becoming a parent
Becoming a parent is one of the major transitions of adult life for both men and women and the stress of not being able to experience this has been associated with a range of psychological problems including anger, depression, anxiety, feelings of defectiveness and incompetence, relationship problems, sexual dysfunction and social isolation [1,2,3]. When you decide to have a baby you step onto a rollercoaster of emotions that doesn't ever really end. Trying to conceive presents you with a raft of emotional challenges, once you conceive you face the challenge of pregnancy and then, when your baby is born you face the challenge of parenting. Learning to better manage your emotions at this stage will therefore benefit you not only now but for the rest of yours and your children's life.

The link between emotional and physical health
Another reason to give this part of your wellbeing attention when you are trying to conceive is that evidence suggests that poor mental health has a detrimental impact on physical health. For example, it has been found that suffering from depression increases your chances of developing heart disease by 67% and cancer by 50% [4]. More specifically one study reported a 2-fold increase in the risk of infertility among women with a history of depressive symptoms [5]. It is thought that depression and anxiety could directly affect fertility by elevating prolactin levels and disrupting the hypothalamic-pituitary-adrenal axis, thyroid and immune function. Depression and anxiety have also been associated with the abnormal regulation of the luteinizing hormone, a hormone that regulates ovulation [6].

Managing your emotions
We have evolved to feel emotions and like all of evolutions creations emotions are fundamental to our existence and survival. Our emotions allow us to navigate through life, enabling us to face challenges, cease opportunities, avoid danger and ensure the ongoing

survival of our species by creating a bond between us and our young allowing us to care, protect and nurture them.

There are 4 main emotions:
Happiness
Anxiety
Anger
Sadness

All other emotions are variations of these four. Identify the emotion(s) that you struggle with the most and go to the section on this emotion for strategies on how to manage it better. Although some people do struggle with happiness, this is usually an indication of a deeper level problem that is likely to need professional support (see section below) and therefore its management is beyond the scope of this book.

Getting more support
If after working through this programme you feel as if you need some additional help to manage the psychological and emotional challenges of trying to conceive a child and becoming a parent a course of Cognitive Behavioural Therapy may be useful for you. Cognitive Behavioural Therapy (CBT) is a talking therapy which equips you with a comprehensive understanding of why you are struggling with an issue and a clear set of psychological and practical tools to resolve this. CBT has a robust evidence base across a range of emotional and physical difficulties including fertility problems. For example, in a study of women who were not ovulating where one group received CBT and the other group was just observed 80% of the women who received CBT started to ovulate again, as opposed to only 25% from the randomized observation group [7].

The British CBT & Counselling Service is a team of Doctors of Clinical and Counselling Psychology specialising in the use of CBT for individuals with fertility problems and the associated psychological and emotional challenges.

For more information on CBT please contact them:
http://www.thebritishcbtcounsellingservice.com/

Anxiety

The function of anxiety is to prepare and motivate us. Without anxiety we would be ill-equipped to face the physical and psychological challenges that life throws at us.

Anxiety and the way we respond when we feel it has evolved to ensure our safety and survival and to optimise our reactions and capabilities. For example, feeling anxious before an exam motivates us to prepare and optimises our performance, feeling anxious in the face of physical danger motivates us to be hypervigilant and wary.

However, although anxiety can be useful in the face of emotional challenges, it is primarily a response to physical challenges. Evolution is a slow process and it has not yet caught up with the way that we currently live our lives i.e. facing many more emotional than physical challenges. The result of this is that we are often ill-equipped when confronted with emotional challenges and our mind and body is forced to fall back on its physical response to stress. So, when trying to conceive we may find our mind and body responding as if we are being chased by a tiger; thoughts of impending doom, feelings of hopelessness and a selection of the intense and uncomfortable physical feelings associated with panic (breathlessness, heart palpitations, dizziness, nausea, confusion).

How to manage your Anxiety
Monitor the fluctuations
Begin by keeping an anxiety diary. Rate the strength of your anxiety on a scale of 0-10 two to three times a day. After a week notice the fluctuations in your anxiety and how, even if your anxiety remains consistently higher, there are still fluctuations within these high scores indicating that there are times when you do not feel as bad.

Identify your thoughts
It is the way that we think about things that determines how we feel about them, positive thoughts lead to positive feelings, negative thoughts to negative feelings etc. Two people in the same situation

can feel very differently and what determines this difference is the way that they think about it.

So, when your anxiety rises above a 6/10 try to identify the thought that preceded/accompanied it. To begin with you may have to go with your best guess as many of our thoughts sit just outside of our conscious awareness. Start with the fact that a combination of 2 types of thoughts are necessary to provoke anxiety and try to identify both types:

1. Overestimating a disaster or catastrophe
   E.g. *I am never going to be a mother*

2. Underestimating your ability to cope
   E.g. *I will never enjoy anything again and will be permanently depressed*

Tip: Try to record your thought in first person, present tense as in the examples above. This makes it easier to complete the exercises outlined below.

Change your Thoughts

Step 1: Define the Worst-Case Scenario

Human beings are hardwired in times of stress to go straight to the worst-case scenario (e.g. *I am never going to be a mother*) and make it the reality. This is a survival strategy: if you are foraging by a bush and it rustles it makes sense to assume the worst (i.e. there is something in there that will eat me) and run, all that is lost is some foraging time. Not assuming the worst could lead to a much more catastrophic outcome. As mentioned above, evolution is a slow process leaving us to deal with many emotional challenges with strategies designed for physical ones, which means we are often ill-equipped in the face of anxiety triggered by fertility challenges. However, this is just our default position and an awareness of this tendency gives us an opportunity to do something different and alleviate the anxiety we feel.

Start by defining your worst case scenario in as much detail as possible so you know exactly what it is that is making you feel anxious, this is the first step to dealing with it.

Step 2: Possibility vs Probability

Most things are possible but when we are anxious we have a tendency to confuse possibility with probability. Look at your worst case scenario and rank its probability (e.g. it has an 5% chance of happening). Remember to be as accurate as possible, basing your assessment on facts not feelings. Accurately assessing the likelihood of your worst case scenario diminishes it's power and will help you to stop overestimating the disaster/catastrophe, the first type of thought that triggers anxiety.

Step 3: Coping with the Worst Case Scenario

If you are able to cope with your worst case scenario, everything else will become the proverbial walk in the park and despite the unlikelihood of it occurring, knowing that you could cope with your worst case scenario diminishes the power of the second type of thought that triggers anxiety; underestimating your ability to cope. So work out how you would deal with the worst case scenario in the unlikely event that it occurs.

Anger

Anger serves an important function, we know this because we all feel it, which suggests that we have evolved to feel it. Anger alerts us to the mistreatment of ourselves (and others). It signals to us when our needs are not being met, needs that have to be met to ensure our physical and psychological wellbeing. Without anger our species would not have been so successful or have survived so long.

However, sometimes we feel angry in the absence of mistreatment, when our needs are not being neglected. Frequently anger becomes the 'go to' when we are experiencing less tolerable emotions, for example, anxiety and sadness, because anger, unlike other emotions, can be projected onto others (it's your fault, not mine) offering us some short-term relief.

In this instance anger becomes the 'cover story' for emotions with more complex origins, so instead of enhancing our experience and ability to function it undermines us by masking the true emotions and the problems at their source.

How to manage Anger
To work out if you are angry or if it is a cover story for another emotion, follow the steps below:

Identify the source of your anger, ask yourself if your needs are being met or if you are being abused or mistreated. If you discover the source of the mistreatment use your anger as a signal to act and resolve this in order to get your needs met, your anger will then dissipate.

If you find that you are not being neglected (which may well be the case if your anger is linked to your fertility challenges), identify the thoughts that directly precede your anger. Then ask yourself whether these thoughts match your feelings, should they trigger anger? Or does it make more sense for them to trigger another emotion (e.g. anxiety, sadness)?

If the thoughts that precede your anger combine an overestimation of some future disaster with an underestimation of your ability to cope with this, your anger is a cover story for anxiety.

If the thoughts that precede your anger involve self-criticism, negative self-evaluation or negative comparison with others, your anger is a cover for depression/sadness.

Anger is a powerful and consuming emotion, it is designed that way to ensure we respond to it and essential needs are met. However, when it is becomes a cover for other emotions it hinders rather than helps us. If you discover that this is the case with your anger, once you have identified the core emotion go to the appropriate section of this document for advice on managing it.

Depression

Depression is the result of self-critical thoughts, a combination of negative evaluations of yourself and negative comparisons with others. If you have a tendency towards self-criticism the challenge of fertility is likely to provoke self-critical thoughts and in turn feelings of depression/sadness. There is no doubt that it is appropriate at times to feel extremely sad if you are struggling to conceive a child, we are hard-wired to feel sadness in such situations of loss or lacking to encourage self-reflection which eventually leads to acceptance and an ability to move forward. However, self-criticism layered on top of what is a functional emotional experience can be tormenting and self-destructive and can spiral into depression.

If you feel you have reached this point, follow the steps below:

1. Identify the thought
The majority of the self-critical thoughts that are responsible for depression sit in our unconscious awareness. This is because our conscious awareness is reserved for new and active thinking e.g. information processing and problem solving. The self-critical thoughts associated with depression have usually been around for some time and so have been relegated to our subconscious to create space for new and active thinking.

This allows our thought processes to be more efficient but it means that the thoughts responsible for problems like depression are sometimes hard to get hold of. However, we cannot deal with something that we aren't aware of, so the first thing we must do when tackling self-critical thoughts is to identify them.

The type of self-critical thoughts that sit in our subconscious occur automatically (i.e. without the need of conscious intervention), so in order to identify them we need to practice focusing on them. This may take a bit of time but by drawing our attention to our thoughts whenever we feel depressed and asking ourselves 'what am I thinking?', we will gradually be able to pull self-critical thoughts into conscious awareness where we can work on them. Bear in mind that self-critical thoughts take the form of negative evaluations of yourself ('I'm not good enough', 'There is something wrong with me') and/or negative comparisons with others ('They are (doing) better than me').

Tip: Record the self-critical thought in first person, present tense as in the examples above as they are easier to work with in this format.

2. Assess accuracy

Once you have identified a self-critical thought assess the accuracy of that thought. For example, are you ignoring important details that may lead to a more positive, accurate or helpful evaluation of yourself or a past event? Has your thinking become black or white; a situation falls short of perfect so you see it as a total failure? Are you seeing a single negative event as a never-ending pattern of defeat by using words such as 'always' or 'never' when you think about it? Are you picking out a single negative detail and dwelling on it exclusively so that your vision of all of reality becomes darkened, like the drop of ink that discolours a beaker of water? Some common thinking patterns that effect the accuracy of our thoughts are listed in the box below.

Thinking Patterns

1. All or nothing - thinking

You see things in black and white categories. If a situation falls short of perfect, you see it as a total failure. When a young woman on a diet ate a spoonful of ice cream, she told herself, 'I've blown my diet completely.' This thought upset her so much that she gobbled down an entire quart of ice cream!

2. Overgeneralization

You see a single negative event, such as a romantic rejection or a career reversal as a never-ending pattern of defeat by using words such as 'always' or 'never' when you think about it. A depressed salesman became terribly upset when he noticed bird dung on the windshield of his car. He told himself, 'Just my luck! Birds are always crapping on my car!'

3. Mental filter

You pick out a single negative detail and dwell on it exclusively, so that your vision of all of reality becomes darkened, like the drop of ink that discolours a beaker of water. Example: You receive many positive comments about your presentation to a group of associates at work, but one of them says something mildly critical. You obsess about his reaction for days and ignore all the positive feedback.

4. Discounting the positive

You reject positive experiences by insisting they 'don't count.' If you do a good job, you may tell yourself that it wasn't good enough or that anyone could have done as well. Discounting the positive takes the joy out of life and makes you feel inadequate and unrewarded.

5. Jumping to conclusions

You interpret things negatively when there are no facts to support your conclusion.

Mind reading: Without checking it out, you arbitrarily conclude that someone is reacting negatively to you.

Fortune telling: You predict that things will turn out badly. Before a test you may tell yourself, 'I'm really going to blow it. What if I flunk?' If you're depressed you may tell yourself, 'I'll never get better.'

6. Magnification

You exaggerate the importance of your problems and shortcomings, or you minimize the importance of your desirable qualities. This is also called the 'binocular trick.'

7. Emotional reasoning

You assume that your negative emotions necessarily reflect the way things really are: 'I feel terrified about going on airplanes. It must be very dangerous to fly.' Or 'I feel guilty. I must be a rotten person.' Or 'I feel angry. This proves I'm being treated unfairly.' Or 'I feel so inferior. This means I'm a second-rate person.' Or 'I feel hopeless. I must really be hopeless.'

Thinking Patterns Cont.

8. "Should statements"

You tell yourself that things should be the way you hoped or expected them to be. After playing a difficult piece on the piano, a gifted pianist told herself, 'I shouldn't have made so many mistakes.' This made her feel so disgusted that she quit practicing for several days. 'Musts,' 'oughts' and 'have tos' are similar offenders.

'Should statements' that are directed against yourself lead to guilt and frustration.

Should statements that are directed against other people or the world in general lead to anger and frustration: 'He shouldn't be so stubborn and argumentative'. Many people try to motivate themselves with shoulds and shouldn'ts, as if they were delinquents who had to be punished before they could be expected to do anything. 'I shouldn't eat that doughnut.' This usually doesn't work because all these shoulds and musts make you feel rebellious and you get the urge to do just the opposite.

9. Labelling

Labelling is an extreme form of all-or-nothing thinking. Instead of saying 'I made a mistake', you attach a negative label to yourself: 'I'm a loser.' You might also label yourself 'a fool' or 'a failure' or 'a jerk.' Labelling is quite irrational because you are not the same as what you do. Human beings exist, but 'fools,' 'losers,' and 'jerks' do not. These labels are useless abstractions that lead to anger, anxiety, frustration, and low self- esteem.

You may also label others. When someone does something that rubs you the wrong way, you may tell yourself: 'He's an S.O.B', then you feel that the problem is with that person's 'character' or 'essence' instead of with their thinking or behaviour. You see them as totally bad. This makes you feel hostile and hopeless about improving things and leaves little room for constructive communication.

10. Personalization

Personalization occurs when you hold yourself personally responsible for an event that isn't entirely under your control. When a woman received a note that her child was having difficulties at school, she told herself, 'this shows what a bad mother I am,' instead of trying to pinpoint the cause of the problem so that she could be helpful to her child. When another woman's husband beat her, she told herself, 'if only I were better in bed, he wouldn't beat me.' Personalization leads to guilt, shame, and feelings of inadequacy.

Some people do the opposite. They blame other people or their circumstances for their problems, and they overlook ways that they might be contributing to the problem: 'The reason my marriage is so lousy is because my spouse is totally unreasonable.' Blame usually doesn't work very well because other people will resent being a scapegoat and they will just toss the blame right back in your lap. It's like the game of hot potato - no one wants to get stuck with it.

3. Assess helpfulness

Sometimes self-critical thoughts are quite accurate but do not give us a helpful way forward. For example, when trying to escape from the top floor of a burning building it may be accurate to think 'I could fall to my death' but it is not a very helpful focus. Something useful can be achieved or learnt from every experience and opportunity but identifying this is a skill that must be learned and practiced. For example, another month that doesn't result in conception can bring you a step closer to your goal by giving you more information about your mind and body and how you need to support yourself.

4. Construct an accurate and helpful alternative thought

Once you have assessed the accuracy and helpfulness of your thoughts try to discover a more accurate and less self-defeating way of thinking about the situation, one that allows you to feel as if you are taking a step forward and gaining something useful from the experience. This will diminish the influence of your self-critical thoughts and allow depression to dissipate. Use the following worksheet to assist you in this process.

Self-Critical Voice Evaluation Sheet

Self-Critical Thought

State in first person, present tense

" .... "

Rate Belief (%)

1 ....(pre worksheet)   2 ....(post worksheet)

Evidence that supports the Self-Critical Voice

....

....

....

....

....

Evidence that contradicts the Self-Critical Voice

Address each of the bullet points above in turn and then add additional contradictory evidence

....

....

....

....

....

Identify a more accurate and/or helpful alternative thought to replace your self-critical thought
Use the information collected above and adopt a nurturing tone that is accepting, kind and non-judgemental. Try to calm and reassure yourself, allow yourself to see the issue from all angles and then help yourself to think clearly to resolve any problem that remains. Imagine you are talking to a good friend.

....

....

....

....

....

....

....

....

....

....

....

....

Meditation

Meditation is a very effective way of creating some distance between you and your distressing thoughts and feelings. It can still the mind and ground you when you are swept away by self-critical or catastrophic thoughts about the future and feelings of hopelessness and helplessness. There is an increasing scientific evidence base supporting its use in alleviating both psychological, emotional and physical health problems.

Meditation should be practiced at least once daily and for between 5-15 minutes, regularity is more important than the length of each individual practice session. You will usually begin to notice the impact of the meditation after 4-6 weeks of daily practice.

Here is a good example of a meditation practice:
https://tinyurl.com/y95noa9f

Section 7: Miscarriage [1,2,3,4]

Unfortunately for many women miscarriage is a part of having a family. With 1 in 3 pregnancies ending in miscarriage most women who have had 2 or more children will have experienced at least one. Miscarriage is nature's way of ensuring the survival of the human race by allowing only the strongest and healthies pregnancies to continue. Unexplained miscarriage is therefore not a sign that something is wrong with us, it is a sign that our bodies are functioning as they should and that next time we are more likely than not to carry a healthy baby to term. And the statistics bear this out:

- Miscarriage is usually a one-time occurrence.

- Most women who miscarry go on to have a healthy pregnancy. Less than 5 percent of women have two consecutive miscarriages, and only 1 percent have three or more consecutive miscarriages.

As we age miscarriage becomes a more likely part of trying to conceive, however, even at 42 years old when it is estimated that 4 out of 5 of a woman's eggs are not viable, this means that at least every 5 months a good one will come along.

Recurrent Miscarriage
Recurrent miscarriage is a term that will usually be used if you have lost 3 or more pregnancies. It is at this point that most medics will begin to investigate the cause of your miscarriages. Up until this point it is usual to be told that you have just been unlucky and to keep trying. There are various causes of recurrent miscarriage, some of which are treatable, these include:

- Chromosomal abnormalities that are repeatedly passed on by one partner
- *Treatment: Referral to geneticist for further testing*

- Hormonal imbalances e.g. Polycystic ovaries, multiple cysts on ovaries
- *Treatment: Both traditional and alternative therapies can offer a way forward here*

- Blood clotting disorders e.g. Systemic Lupus Rrythematosus and Antiphospholipid Syndrome which cause 'sticky blood'
- *Treatment: Aspirin or Heparin therapy to thin the blood*

- Abnormally shaped womb
- *Treatment: Surgery in some cases*

- Cervical weakness
- *Treatment: A stitch or cervical cerclage early in the pregnancy*

For some couples no cause is ever identified, however 60-70% of women who have had repeated and unexplained miscarriages go on to have healthy pregnancies.

A study published in the journal PLoS ONE offers a different way of thinking about recurrent miscarriage that may enable some couples to continue a little longer on their journey to conceive a child naturally. The study suggests that some women's wombs are too good at letting embryos implant and will accept all embryos including the poor quality ones that other women would reject. The study concludes that in these cases 'super fertility' is responsible for unexplained recurrent miscarriage. So, while a woman with a more selective womb may have to wait 18 months to conceive, a 'super fertile' woman may conceive multiple times during that period and miscarry on each occasion. Both women may eventually carry a healthy baby to term, but each experiences a different kind of pain and frustration along the way.

This research could help women experiencing recurrent miscarriage attach a different meaning to their experience, instead of 'there's something wrong with me' they could think 'my body is too good at this'. As discussed in this book in an earlier chapter looking at emotional wellbeing, the meaning that we attach to things determines how we feel about things and how we feel about things determines the ease with which we are able to cope with them.

Pregnancy After Miscarriage
Pregnancy after a miscarriage is always a challenge, but there are a number of ways to ease your anxiety that history will repeat itself.
Keep in mind everything that we have discussed in this chapter so far, re-read it as often as is helpful, particularly the fact that things are more likely to be okay than not.

Use the tools in the Emotional Wellbeing chapter of this book to help you keep your anxiety and other emotions at a manageable level.
Take one day at a time and try to distract yourself as much as you can by filling your time with activities that give you a sense of achievement and enjoyment.

Keep your mind focused on what is happening now and try to resist the urge to make predictions about what might happen in the future, particularly catastrophic ones. To keep your mind present practice meditation (see chapter on Emotional Wellbeing) which research has shown to be extremely helpful in managing distress and other negative emotions.

If you find statistics helpful this day by day miscarriage risk chart may help you to manage your count down.
https://tinyurl.com/jfryr5d

Section 8: Conceiving Over 35

There is a lot written about the accelerated decline in fertility once a woman passes 35, however, much of this has been overstated:

1. The data upon which much of the citations regarding the accelerated decline in fertility are based have been sourced from church birth records in rural France between 1670 and 1830 when life expectancy was shorter and modern medicine, antibiotics and indoor plumbing amongst other things, didn't exist [1]. Most data on fertility after 40 quoted online (and even in patient guides by doctors) comes from IVF fertility treatment records.

2. The commonly quoted statistic that the chance of pregnancy per cycle is only 5% at age 40 appears to have no original source which places a huge question mark over its reliability [2].

3. A more recent study (1990) found [2] 50% of 35-39 year olds were pregnant after 3 months of trying to conceive, 82% within a year and 90% after 2 years.

4. Having sex 2 days before ovulation led to pregnancy in 25% of 35-39 year olds after 1 cycle whilst 25% of women aged 19-26yrs became pregnant when they had sex 3 days before ovulation. Timing sex better eliminated the age difference in fertility.

5. Historical birth records show that 44% of 40yr olds got pregnant in a year and 64% within 4 years [2].

6. A 1985 study found that among women 40 or older who had at least one child, 36% had a baby within 3 months of

stopping birth control, 59% got pregnant within 9 months, 68% within 18 months and 78% within two years [3].

7. A 2013 study found that among white women ages 40-43 who had at least one child, 60% got pregnant within 6 months [2].

8. Recent studies [4,5] of embryos in IVF cycles found that only 16% of embryos are normal among women aged 40 to 42, and only 8% among those 43 or older. It is not clear if these statistics apply to women trying to conceive naturally. However, even if they do, 16% is 1 out of 6, which would means an average time to get pregnant would be 6 months. However, it could be quicker if you assume that getting a normal embryo is random, the statistics are the same as rolling a 6 on a 6-sided dice. By 4 rolls, more than 50% of people will have rolled a 6.

9. In the 1920s the average age that a woman gave birth to her last child was 42 [2]. It is the baby boomers that have skewed our perception on age and fertility.

10. In the past, it has been thought that we are born with all of the egg cells we will have for the rest of our lives, hence the reason age can have such an impact on egg health. Recent research [6] however has found that women may produce eggs throughout their reproductive years and scientists have found stem cells within the ovaries that produce new egg cells. This is not to say that age does not have an impact on new eggs as the ovaries continue to age, meaning that over time the "housing" for our eggs becomes less than optimal. However, you can protect the eggs you currently have as well as encouraging ovarian health through diet, herbs, supplements and increased circulation to the reproductive system.

11. Both environmental and genetic factors contribute to depletion of the egg pool and reduction in egg quality,

meaning that biological and chronological ovarian age are not always equivalent. So, even if you are a bit older and/or your mother went through the menopause before 45 (often cited as the most influential factor in declining fertility), this is only half the story. Your chronological age can be manipulated through diet, lifestyle and Chinese medicine. Furthermore, biological age is more important than chronological age in predicting the outcome of Assisted Reproductive Technology [7,8].

12. A study published in The Lancet (1991)[9] to ascertain the actual cause of infertility in females over 40 years (mean age of 42.0 years) concluded that ovum related issues are the primary cause of infertility and if normal ovarian cycle is restored, the female reproductive organs in 40 year olds are competent to bear the pregnancy. These conclusions were confirmed in a second study (Human Reproduction, 2002) [10] which looked at women between 41 to 46 years. This second study also suggested that it is the decline in hormonal secretion in women with advancing age that interferes with normal ovulation. This is further complemented by a substantial decrease in the total number of viable oocytes. These factors contribute to the difficulty in conception seen in older women.

Research data clearly suggests that the restoration of a normal balance in female reproductive hormones can help improve fertility rate and chances of conception. Thus the identification and prompt management of factors that may produce an imbalance in the production or metabolism of female hormones becomes an important factor in increasing the chances of conception.

13. IVF favours younger women as it works best if the ovaries produce a lot of eggs at once and as this is less likely if you're older the data here is less encouraging. However, don't be discouraged, if you can rule out tubal and sperm issues, your best chance of conceiving is naturally.

The further past 35 you are the longer it may take you to get pregnant so use the wisdom those extra years have given you to measure your expectations, cultivate patience and most importantly, do not lose hope just because it is taking longer than you would like. There is a saying in the yogic tradition: *When you plant a seed don't constantly scratch the soil to see the sprout.*

Following the plan outlined in this book will maximise your chances of conceiving and will make it more likely than not that you will have a baby.

If you are over 35 and have Polycystic Ovarian Syndrome (PCOS)
A recent study at Uppsala University in Sweden [11] found that women with PCOS not only have roughly the same amount of spontaneous pregnancies as those without the syndrome but that their rates of miscarriage are not increased. The research concludes that this is due to 2 factors. Firstly, women with PCOS may begin life with more eggs than those without which means that as they age, women with PCOS have more eggs left over than those without PCOS. Secondly, ovarian aging naturally results in follicle loss which means that the extra follicles that interfered with the hormonal activity of a woman with PCOS when she was younger will lessen, if not disappear as she ages. This may explain the normalised menstruation cycles reported by some older women with PCOS. So, as women with PCOS age they have more eggs remaining than their non PCOS peers and a more optimal number of follicles in their youth which allows them to 'catch up' in terms of their fertility potential.

References

Introduction

1. http://www.resolve.org/about/fast-facts-about-fertility.html?referrer=https://www.google.co.uk/

2. http://www.marchofdimes.org/volunteers/12-month-pregnancy-program.aspx

Chapter 1

1. http://www.foresight-preconception.org.uk/

2. Rzymski P et al. (2015). Impact of heavy metals on the female reproductive system. Ann Agric Environ Med. https://www.ncbi.nlm.nih.gov/pubmed/26094520

3. Barański M. et al (2014). Higher antioxidant and lower cadmium concentrations and lower incidence of pesticide residues in organically grown crops: a systematic literature review and meta-analyses. British Journal of Nutrition: https://www.cambridge.org/core/journals/british-journal-of-nutrition/article/div-classtitlehigher-antioxidant-and-lower-cadmium-concentrations-and-lower-incidence-of-pesticide-residues-in-organically-grown-crops-a-systematic-literature-review-and-meta-analysesdiv/33F09637EAE6C4ED119E0C4BFFE2D5B1

4. http://www.medicaldaily.com/eating-avocados-more-triples-ivf-pregnancy-success-rate-241240

5. Pandey SK. et al. (2005). Effect of Asparagus racemosus rhizome (Shatavari) on mammary gland and genital organs of pregnant rat. Phytother Res: https://www.ncbi.nlm.nih.gov/pubmed/16177978

6. Wang, J. G. et al. (2007). The effect of cinnamon extract on insulin resistance parameters in polycystic ovary syndrome: a pilot study. *Fertility and sterility*: http://www.fertstert.org/article/S0015-0282%2806%2904555-9/abstract

7. Gonzales GF. et al. (2012). Ethnobiology and Ethnopharmacology of Lepidium meyenii (Maca), a Plant from the Peruvian Highlands. Evid Based Complement Alternat Med: https://www.ncbi.nlm.nih.gov/pmc/articles/PMC3184420/

8. Durairajanayagam D. et al. (2014). Lycopene and male infertility. Asian J Androl: https://www.ncbi.nlm.nih.gov/pmc/articles/PMC4023371/

9. Robbins WA. et al (2012). Walnuts improve semen quality in men consuming a Western-style diet: randomized control dietary intervention trial. Biology of Reproduction: http://www.biolreprod.org/content/87/4/101

10. http://www.acog.org/About-ACOG/News-Room/News-Releases/2013/High-Protein-Low-Carb-Diets-Greatly-Improve-Fertility

11a. Chavarro J.E. et al. (2008). Protein intake and ovulatory infertility. Am J Obstet Gynecol: https://www.ncbi.nlm.nih.gov/pmc/articles/PMC3066040/

11b. https://www.ncbi.nlm.nih.gov/pmc/articles/PMC3074428/

12. Sasikumar S. et al. (2014). A study on significant biochemical changes in the serum of infertile women. *Res. Aca. Rev:* http://www.ijcrar.com/vol-2-2/S.Sasikumar,%20et%20al.pdf

13. Afeiche M. et al. (2013). Meat intake and semen parameters among men attending a fertility clinic. Fertilty and Sterility: http://www.fertstert.org/article/S0015-0282(13)02544-2/fulltext

14. Saldeen. et al (2004). Women and omega-3 fatty acids. Omega-3 FA can facilitate pregnancy in women with infertility problems by increasing uterine blood flow Obstetrical & gynecological survey: https://www.ncbi.nlm.nih.gov/pubmed/15385858

15. Bhathena SJ. et al (1991). Effects of omega 3 fatty acids and vitamin E on hormones involved in carbohydrate and lipid metabolism in men. Carbohydrate Nutrition Laboratory: https://www.ncbi.nlm.nih.gov/pubmed/1832814

16a. Dietary Reference Intakes (DRIs): Recommended Intakes for Energy, Carbohydrate, Fibre, Fat, Fatty Acids, Cholesterol, Protein and Amino Acids (2002) (2005), The National Academies Press.

b. Riccardi G. (2008). Role of glycemic index and glycemic load in the healthy state, in prediabetes, and in diabetes. *American Journal of Clinical Nutrition*, Vol. 87 (1) 269S-274S.

c. http://journals.sagepub.com/doi/abs/10.1177/011542650802300163

17. Maconochie N. et al. (2006). Risk factors for first trimester miscarriage - results from a UK-population-based case-control study. Department of Epidemiology and Population Health, London School of Hygiene & Tropical Medicine, London, UK, BJOG: http://www.lshtm.ac.uk/pressoffice/press_releases/2006/miscarriage.html#sthash.mTcKfK6T.dpuf

18. Pandey S. (2010).The impact of female obesity on the outcome of fertility treatment. J Hum Reprod Sci: https://www.ncbi.nlm.nih.gov/pmc/articles/PMC2970793/

19. Fort P. et al (1990). J. Am. Coll. Nutr. 9 (1990), p. 164

20. Doerge D. et al. (2002). Inactivation of thyroid peroxidase by soy isoflavones in vitro and in vivo. Journal of Chromatography B Vol. 77

21. https://www.newscientist.com/article/dn11266-tubs-of-ice-cream-help-women-make-babies/

22. http://www.fertilityafter40.com/traditional-chinese-medicine--herbs-for-fertility.html

23. Messina M. et al (2206). Effects of soy protein and soybean isoflavones on thyroid function in healthy adults and hypothyroid patients: a review of the relevant literature. Thyroid.16(3):249-58: https://www.ncbi.nlm.nih.gov/pubmed/16571087

24. Carwile J L. (2013). Consumption of Low-Fat Dairy Products May Delay Natural Menopause J Nutr. 143(10): 1642–1650: https://www.ncbi.nlm.nih.gov/pmc/articles/PMC3771815/

25. Hammami I. (2013). Impact of garlic feeding (Allium sativum) on male fertility. Andrologia; 45(4):217-24: https://www.ncbi.nlm.nih.gov/pubmed/22943423

26a. Haas, E. & Levin, B. (2006). Foods. In Staying Healthy with Nutrition; The Complete Guide to Diet and Nutritional Medicine (21st-Century Edition ed.). Berkeley, CA: Celestial Arts.

b. http://www.sciencedirect.com/science/article/pii/S1047279710001213

27. http://www.acupuncturetoday.com/mpacms/at/article.php?id=32643

28. Ly, C. (2014). The effects of dietary polyphenols on reproductive health and early development Hum Reprod Update, 21 (2): 228-248: https://academic.oup.com/humupd/article/21/2/228/783906/The-effects-of-dietary-polyphenols-on-reproductive

29. Sharma R. et al. (2013). Lifestyle factors and reproductive health: taking control of your fertility. Reprod Biol Endocrinol; 11: 66: https://www.ncbi.nlm.nih.gov/pmc/articles/PMC3717046/

30. http://www.livestrong.com/article/523480-how-important-is-drinking-water-to-getting-pregnant/

31. http://www.fertility-health.com/how-much-water-to-drink.html

32. Chavarro JE. (2007). Dietary fatty acid intakes and the risk of ovulatory infertility. Am J Clin Nutr.;85(1):231-7: https://www.ncbi.nlm.nih.gov/pubmed/17209201

33. http://www.dietinpregnancy.co.uk/pregnancy/caffeine-pregnancy.html

34. Eggert J. (2004). Effects of alcohol consumption on female fertility during an 18-year period. Fertil Steril.Feb;81(2):379-83: https://www.ncbi.nlm.nih.gov/pubmed/14967377

35. Jenson, TK. (1998). Does moderate alcohol consumption affect fertility? Follow up study among couples planning first pregnancy. BMJ. Aug 22; 317(7157): 505–510: https://www.ncbi.nlm.nih.gov/pmc/articles/PMC28642/

36.https://dash.harvard.edu/bitstream/handle/1/27336535/nihms6993 11.pdf?sequence=1

37. http://www.nhs.uk/news/2014/10October/Pages/Moderate-regular-drinking-may-still-damage-sperm.aspx

38. Götz F. (2001). Female infertility--effect of perinatal xenoestrogen exposure on reproductive functions in animals and humans. Folia Histochem Cytobiol.;39 Suppl 2:40-3: https://www.ncbi.nlm.nih.gov/pubmed/11820621

39. http://news.bbc.co.uk/1/hi/health/2276733.stm

40. Bast A. et al (2209). Celiac Disease and Reproductive Health. Practical Gastroenterology: http://natural-fertility-info.com/wp-content/uploads/BastArticle.pdf

41. Aguiar F.M., et. al. (2009). "Serological testing for celiac disease in women with endometriosis. A pilot study". Clin. Exp. Obstet. Gynecol. 36 (1), 23-25. http://europepmc.org/abstract/med/19400413

42. https://www.coeliac.org.uk/coeliac-disease/associated-conditions-and-complications/fertility-problems/

43. http://www.drdavidwilliams.com/gut-health-and-the-benefits-of-traditional-fermented-foods/

44. http://www.bbcgoodfood.com/howto/guide/health-benefits-offermenting

45. http://www.foodandnutrition.org/Winter-2012/The-History-and-Health-Benefits-of-Fermented-Food/

Chapter 2

1. http://www.medicalnewstoday.com/articles/301350.php

2. http://www.medicinesinpregnancy.org/Medicine--pregnancy/Asprin/

3. Buhling KJ. (2013). The effect of micronutrient supplements on female fertility. Curr Opin Obstet Gynecol.;25(3):173-80: https://www.ncbi.nlm.nih.gov/pubmed/23571830

4. Watanabe T. (2003). The effects of dietary vitamin B12 deficiency on sperm maturation in developing and growing male rats. Congenit Anom (Kyoto). 2003 Mar;43(1):57-64; https://www.ncbi.nlm.nih.gov/pubmed/12692404

5. Nutrients and Vitamins for Pregnancy: American Pregnancy Association. (2012, April 26): http://americanpregnancy.org/pregnancy-health/nutrients-vitamins-pregnancy/

6. http://www.marilynglenville.com/womens-health-issues/infertility/

7. Henmi, H. et al. (2003). Effects of ascorbic acid supplementation on serum progesterone levels in patients with a luteal phase defect. *Fertility and sterility*, 80(2), 459-461: https://www.ncbi.nlm.nih.gov/pubmed/12909517

8. Akmal M. (2006). Improvement in human semen quality after oral supplementation of vitamin C;9(3):440-2: https://www.ncbi.nlm.nih.gov/pubmed/17004914

9. http://www.whitelotusclinic.ca/blog/dr-fiona-nd/natural-treatments-for-autoimmune-infertility-concerns/

9b. Pal L. et al. (2012). Therapeutic implications of vitamin D and calcium in overweight women with polycystic ovary syndrome. Gynecological Endocrinology, 28(12), pp.965-968.

10. Takasaki A. et al. (2010) Endometrial growth and uterine blood flow: a pilot study for improving endometrial thickness in the patients with a thin endometrium. *Fertil. Steril.* 93 (6): 1851–8: https://www.ncbi.nlm.nih.gov/pubmed/19200982

11. Keskes-Ammar L.et al.(2003). Sperm oxidative stress and the effect of an oral vitamin E and selenium supplement on semen quality in infertile men. *Systems Biology in Reproductive Medicine*, 49(2), 83-94: https://www.ncbi.nlm.nih.gov/pmc/articles/PMC3988936/

12. http://www.nhs.uk/Conditions/Spina-bifida/Pages/Causes.aspx

13. http://www.altmedrev.com/publications/7/6/512.pdf

14. Lenzi, Andrea, M.D., et al. (2004) A placebo-controlled double-blind randomized trial of the use of combined L-carnitine and L-acetyl-carnitine treatment in men with asthenozoospermia. *Fertility*

and Sterility p. 1578–1584, Vol. 81, Issue 6, June:
https://www.ncbi.nlm.nih.gov/pubmed/15193480

15. Lenzi, Andrea, M.D., et al. (2003) Use of carnitine therapy in selected cases of male factor infertility: a double-blind crossover trial. *Fertility and Sterility* p. 292–300, Vol. 79, No. 2, February: https://www.ncbi.nlm.nih.gov/pubmed/12568837

16. http://www.livescience.com/17878-dha-vital-sperm-health.html

17. Simopoulos AP. (2002). The importance of the ratio of omega-6/omega-3 essential fatty acids. Biomedecine & Pharmacotherapy Volume 56, Issue 8:
https://www.ncbi.nlm.nih.gov/pubmed/12442909.

18. Saldeen P et al. (2004) Women and omega-3 fatty acids. Omega-3 FA can facilitate pregnancy in women with infertility problems by increasing uterine blood flow Obstetrical & gynecological survey, vol. 59, no10: https://www.ncbi.nlm.nih.gov/pubmed/15385858

19. Sieve BF. (1942). The clinical effects of a new B-complex factor, para-aminobenzoic acid, on pigmentation and fertility. *South Med Surg* (March);104:135-139.

a. Moslemi MK. (2011). Selenium–vitamin E supplementation in infertile men: effects on semen parameters and pregnancy rate. Int J Gen Med; 4: 99–104:
https://www.ncbi.nlm.nih.gov/pmc/articles/PMC3048346/

b. Amar E. et al (2015). Treatment for High Levels of Sperm DNA Fragmentation and Nuclear De condensation: Sequential Treatment with a Potent Antioxidant Followed by Stimulation of the One-Carbon Cycle vs One-Carbon Cycle Back-up Alone. Austin Journal of Reproductive Medicine and Infertility.

20. Dantillo M. et al (2014). The importance of the one carbon cycle nutritional support in human male fertility: a preliminary clinical report. Reproductive Biology and Endocrinology, 12:71

21. Ebisch IM, et al. The importance of folate, zinc and antioxidants in the pathogenesis and prevention of subfertility. Hum Reprod Update. 2007 Mar-Apr;13(2):163-74:
https://www.ncbi.nlm.nih.gov/pubmed/17099205

22. Zhao J. et al. (2016). Zinc levels in seminal plasma and their correlation with male infertility: A systematic review and meta-analysis. Sci Rep; 6: 22386:
https://www.ncbi.nlm.nih.gov/pmc/articles/PMC4773819/

23. www.biomedcentral.com/content/pdf/1477-7827-9-23.pdf

24. Ben-Meir A. et al. (2015). CoQ10 treatment can improve fertility and oocyte quality in old mice. Fertility and Sterility Vol. 96, Issue 3:
https://www.ncbi.nlm.nih.gov/pubmed/26111777

25. Balercia G. et al. (2009). Coenzyme Q10 and male infertility. J Endocrinol Invest ;32(7):626-32:
https://www.ncbi.nlm.nih.gov/pubmed/19509475

26. https://www.centerforhumanreprod.com/services/infertility-treatments/

27. https://www.chronobiology.com/the-role-of-melatonin-in-fertility-and-conception/

28. Kamel HH. (20130. Role of phyto-oestrogens in ovulation induction in women with polycystic ovarian syndrome. Eur J Obstet Gynecol Reprod Biol:
https://www.ncbi.nlm.nih.gov/pubmed/23347605

29. http://www.aafp.org/afp/2005/0901/p821.html

30. Unfer V. et al (2012). Effects of myo-inositol in women with PCOS: a systematic review of randomized controlled trials. Gynecol Endocrinol;28(7):509-15:
https://www.ncbi.nlm.nih.gov/pubmed/22296306

31. Saha L. et al. (2013). *N*-acetyl cysteine in clomiphene citrate resistant polycystic ovary syndrome: A review of reported outcomes. J Pharmacol Pharmacother; 4(3): 187–191: https://www.ncbi.nlm.nih.gov/pmc/articles/PMC3746301/

32. Qin B. etal . (2010). Cinnamon: Potential Role in the Prevention of Insulin Resistance, Metabolic Syndrome, and Type 2 Diabetes. J Diabetes Sci Technol; 4(3): 685–693: https://www.ncbi.nlm.nih.gov/pmc/articles/PMC2901047/

33. Henmi H. et al. (2003). Effects of ascorbic acid supplementation on serum progesterone levels in patients with a luteal phase defect. *Fertility and Sterility*, 80(2), 459-461: https://www.ncbi.nlm.nih.gov/pubmed/12909517

34. Agarwal A. et al. (2005). Role of oxidative stress in female reproduction. *Reprod Biol Endocrinol*, 3(28), 1-21: https://www.ncbi.nlm.nih.gov/pubmed/16018814

Chapter 3

1. Twenge J. (2012). The Impatient Woman's Guide to Getting Pregnant. Atria Paperback: New York.

2. Stirnemann JJ. (2013). Day-specific probabilities of conception in fertile cycles resulting in spontaneous pregnancies. Hum Reprod;28(4): https://www.ncbi.nlm.nih.gov/pubmed/23340057

3. Barrett JC. (1967). The risk of conception on different days of the menstrual cycle. Population Studies, 23, 455.

4. Dunson DB. et al. (1999). Day-specific probabilities of clinical pregnancy based on two studies with imperfect measures of ovulation. Human Reproduction, 14, 1835-1839.

5. Dunson DB. et al (2002). Changes with age in the level and duration of fertility in the menstrual cycle. Human Reproduction, 17, 1399-1403.

6. Stanford JB. et al (2007). Effect of sexual intercourse patterns in time to pregnancy studies. American Journal of Epidemiology, 165, 1088-1095.

7. Stanford JB. et al (2002). Timing intercourse to achieve pregnancy: Current evidence. Obstetrics & Gynecology, 100, 1333-1341.

8. https://www.cmu.edu/CSR/case_studies/passionate_sex.html

9. Custers IM. (2009). Immobilisation versus immediate mobilisation after intrauterine insemination. British Medical Journal, 339, b4080.

10. http://natural-fertility-info.com/mens-fertility

11. http://www.pcrm.org/health/reports/diet-fertility-and-sperm-count

12. Erik O. (1968) The Functional Structure of Human Cervical Mucus. Acta Obstetricia et Gynecologica Scandinavica, Volume 47, Issue S1

13. Katz DF. et al. (1978). The movement of human spermatozoa in cervical mucus. *Journal of Reproduction and Fertility*; Vol 53 259-265

14. Gorodeski GI. (2000). NO increases permeability of cultured human cervical epithelia by cGMP-mediated increase in G-actin. *Am J Physiol* Cell Physiol 278: C942-C952

15. Weschler T. (2002). Taking charge of your fertility. Harper Collins: United States

16. http://americanpregnancy.org/getting-pregnant/track-ovulation-irregular-periods/

17. http://www.whattoexpect.com/preconception/fertility/five-ways-to-tell-you-are-ovulating.aspx

18.https://www.fertilityfriend.com/landing.html?gclid=CNi9uovSodI CFQEA0wodFvYI3w

Chapter 4

1. http://www.fitnessmagazine.com/health/pregnancy/how-exercise-affects-fertility/

2. http://www.nhs.uk/news/2009/11November/Pages/get-fit-exercise-infertility-problems.aspx

3. https://www.ncbi.nlm.nih.gov/pubmed/7127652

4. https://www.fitpregnancy.com/pregnancy/getting-pregnant/how-get-pregnant

5. https://www.tcmworld.org/programs/womens-health/pre-and-post-pregnancy/

6. http://www.pullingdownthemoon.com/blog/2012/february/annas-news-appropriate-exercise-according-to-chi.aspx

7. http://www.nychi-acupuncture.com/blog/the-menstrual-cycle-according-to-traditional-chinese-medicine/

8.http://www.reproductivefacts.org/uploadedFiles/ASRM_Content/R esources/Patient_Resources/Fact_Sheets_and_Info_Booklets/smokin g.pdf

9. https://www.ncbi.nlm.nih.gov/pubmed/8885914

10.http://www.nhs.uk/Livewell/Fertility/Pages/Protectyourfertility.aspx

11. https://www.ncbi.nlm.nih.gov/pmc/articles/PMC4402098/

12. https://www.rrc.com/how-lack-of-sleep-is-hurting-your-fertility/

13. http://natural-fertility-info.com/problems-sleeping-hormonal-balance.html

Chapter 5

1. https://nccih.nih.gov/health/whatiscam/chinesemed.htm

2. http://natural-fertility-info.com/how-traditional-chinese-medicine-acupuncture-enhances-fertility

3. http://rchm.co.uk/what-is-chinese-herbal-medicine/

4. https://www.tcmworld.org/

5. http://www.itmonline.org/arts/fertility.htm

6. https://www.ncbi.nlm.nih.gov/pmc/articles/PMC3388479/

7. https://nccih.nih.gov/research/results/spotlight/072913

8.http://www.nhs.uk/news/2007/January08/Pages/AcupunctureandsuccessofIVF.aspx

9. http://www.acupuncture.org.uk/a-to-z-of-conditions/a-to-z-of-conditions/female-fertility.html

10. http://www.webmd.com/infertility-and-reproduction/features/ancient-art-of-infertility-treatment#1

11. https://www.jcm.co.uk/

12. http://www.pullingdownthemoon.com/blog/2015/october/study-finds-significant-benefits-of-yoga-for-wom.aspx

13. http://www.yogajournal.com/article/health/fertile-ground/

14. https://www.ncbi.nlm.nih.gov/pmc/articles/PMC3733210/

15. http://www.yogajournal.com/category/health/fertility/

16. http://natural-fertility-info.com/fertility-massage

17. http://naturalhealthbag.com/fertility-massage-self-massage-techniques-uterus-ovary/

18. http://www.natural-health-for-fertility.com/massage-for-fertility.html

19.http://www.bbc.co.uk/devon/community_life/features/ivf_reflexol ogy.shtml

20. http://natural-fertility-info.com/castor-oil-therapy

21. http://www.springmoonfertility.com/castor-oil-packs/

22. http://lunaception.net/

23. http://www.naturalfertilityandwellness.com/basics-of-charting-and-lunaception/

24. http://www.motherrisingbirth.com/2015/11/lunaception.html

Chapter 6

1. http://www.bestpracticeobgyn.com/article/S1521-6934(06)00161-1/abstract?cc=y=

2. http://www.tandfonline.com/doi/abs/10.1300/J010v11n04_05

3. http://www.tandfonline.com/doi/abs/10.3109/00016341003623746

4. https://www.mentalhealth.org.uk/a-to-z/p/physical-health-and-mental-health

5. http://www.bjmp.org/content/psychological-aspects-infertility

6. https://academic.oup.com/humrep/article/16/7/1420/693403/The-effect-of-anxiety-and-depression-on-the

7. http://news.bbc.co.uk/1/hi/health/5098454.stm

Chapter 7

1. http://www.miscarriageassociation.org.uk/

2. http://www.nhs.uk/Conditions/Miscarriage/Pages/Introduction.aspx

3. https://www.tommys.org/our-organisation/why-we-exist/miscarriage-statistics

4. Weimar C.H.E. et al (2012) Endometrial Stromal Cells of Women with Recurrent Miscarriage Fail to Discriminate between High- and Low-Quality Human Embryos. PLOS ONE: http://journals.plos.org/plosone/article?id=10.1371/journal.pone.0041424

Chapter 8

1. Dunson, D. B. et al (2002). Changes with age in the level and duration of fertility in the menstrual cycle. Human Reproduction, 17, 1399-1403.

2. Twenge, J.M. (2013). The Impatient Woman's Guide to Getting Pregnant.

3. Menken, J. et al (1986). Age and infertility. Science, 26, 1389-1394.

4. Belloc, S. (2008). Effect of maternal and paternal age on pregnancy and miscarriage rates after intrauterine insemination. Reproductive BioMedicine Online, 17, 392-97.

5. Klipstein, S. et al (2005). One last chance for pregnancy: A review of 2,705 in vitro fertilization cycles initiated in women age 40 years and above. Fertility and Sterility, 84, 435-45.

6. http://www.nature.com/news/egg-making-stem-cells-found-in-adult-ovaries-1.10121

7. https://rbej.biomedcentral.com/articles/10.1186/1477-7827-7-101

8. https://www.ncbi.nlm.nih.gov/pmc/articles/PMC3843177/

9. https://www.ncbi.nlm.nih.gov/pubmed/1674764

10.https://academic.oup.com/humrep/article/17/12/3065/569578/Serum-anti-Mullerian-hormone-levels-a-novel

11. https://www.researchgate.net/publication/23939186_Long-term_follow-up_of_patients_with_polycystic_ovary_syndrome_Reproductive_outcome_and_ovarian_reserve

About the Author

I am a Doctor of Clinical Psychology specialising in helping couples overcome the challenges of fertility and parenting. Over the last 16 years I have helped hundreds of couples through the process of conception, pregnancy, birth and the early years of parenting using a combination of evidence based techniques to optimise physical and psychological health.

I trained for 9 years first at the University of Exeter and then at the University of East London. I went on to work as a Consultant Clinical Psychologist for 7 years in the NHS during which time I ran a specialist service offering Cognitive Behavioural Therapy (CBT) and published widely in the field of Psychology. I have also spoken at numerous national and international conferences on the topic of Cognitive Behavioural Therapy (CBT). In 2001 I set up The British CBT & Counselling Service, a national private psychology service offering individually tailored CBT and counselling programmes to adults and children with a range of mental health problems. I continue to work here as the Clinical Lead of a team of Doctors of Clinical and Counselling Psychology.

At the age of 19 years I was diagnosed with a severe case of Polycystic Ovarian Syndrome (PCOS) and as a result suffered from amenorrhoea (a lack of menstrual periods) throughout my twenties and early thirties. I was told by specialists that it was unlikely that I would be able to have children. However, by following the programme outlined in this book I was able to establish a regular menstrual cycle and had my first child at the age of 35. I went on to have two more children at 36 and 39 years. As I write this book I am pregnant with my fourth child who is due a week before my 44th birthday.

All of my children have been conceived naturally and within a few months of trying to conceive. Between my third and fourth child I experienced 3 consecutive miscarriages in less than a year. I mention this to demonstrate the fact that miscarriage is a common and normal part of conception and pregnancy and rarely a sign that you will not eventually have a baby.